Pocket Guide to Lung Cancer

Jones and Bartlett Series in Oncology

Pocket Guide to Lung Cancer

Marilyn Haas, PhD, RN, CNS, ANP-C

Mountain Radiation Oncology
Asheville, North Carolina

JONES AND BARTLETT PUBLISHERS
Sudbury, Massachusetts
BOSTON   TORONTO   LONDON   SINGAPORE

World Headquarters

Jones and Bartlett
  Publishers
40 Tall Pine Drive
Sudbury, MA 01776
978-443-5000
info@jbpub.com
www.jbpub.com

Jones and Bartlett
  Publishers Canada
2406 Nikanna Road
Mississauga,
  ON L5C 2W6
CANADA

Jones and Bartlett
  Publishers
  International
Barb House, Barb
  Mews
London W6 7PA
UK

Acquisitions Editor: Penny M. Glynn
Production Manager: Amy Rose
Editorial Assistant: Amy Sibley
Production Assistant: Tracey Chapman
Marketing Manager: Joy Stark-Vancs
Marketing Associate: Elizabeth Waterfall
Manufacturing and Inventory Coordinator: Amy Bacus
Cover Design: Bret Kerr
Composition: Dartmouth Publishing, Inc.
Printing and Binding: United Graphics
Cover Printing: United Graphics

Printed in the United States of America
07 06 05 04 03   10 9 8 7 6 5 4 3 2 1

Dedication

"Far away there in the sunshine are my highest aspirations, I may not reach them, but I can look up and see their beauty, believe in them, and try to follow where they lead."

While unable to provide recognition to the author of this quote, the support I have from my lung cancer patients, colleagues, friends, and family (Bill, William, and Kenneth) never goes unrecognized. Without their support, my aspirations would never become realities.

Contents

Disclaimer

Technological explosions have impacted the area of oncology, from the diagnostic tests and pharmacological agents to the equipment available to treat individuals with lung cancer. While research is being conducted by many organizations, healthcare providers are still searching for the best evidence medicine. The information provided in this pocket guide is in accord with recommendations at the time of publication, and every effort was made to ensure accuracy. However, before administering any drug, the reader is advised to check the manufacturer's product information sheet for the most current recommendations on dosage, precautions, contraindications, and potential side effects. This also holds true for any diagnostic testing/imaging. The reader is advised that the authors, editors, reviewers, and publisher cannot be responsible for any errors or omissions in this guide, or for any resulting consequences.

Preface

The *Pocket Guide to Lung Cancer* is a quick reference that oncology professionals can refer to at a glance. This guide supplements the *Contemporary Issues in Lung Cancer* textbook, and provides clinical information that supports oncology professionals caring for the patient with lung cancer. While some of the information at the beginning aligns with the textbook (Parts I and II contain updated information added to each chapter), Parts III and IV are new sections. The abbreviated clinical notes in Part III, the symptom management/intervention section, will provide initial recommendations to care for the patient undergoing treatment. Certainly, it is not intended as an exhaustive compilation of all available interventions, but should be utilized as a reference point. Part IV will assist in patient education.

Acknowledgments

The *Contemporary Issues in Lung Cancer* came to fruition because many experts were willing to research and share their knowledge and clinical expertise in caring for lung cancer patients. It is my pleasure to again thank them for their input:

Pamela M. Calarese, RN, MS, CS
Patricia A. Carter, RN, PhD, CNS
Cynthia Chernecky, RN, PhD, AOCN
Mary E. Cooley, PhD, CRNP
Doris Dickerson Coward, RN, PhD
Marianne J. Davies, RN, MSN, OCN, APRN, ACNP
L. Tammy Duckworth, MA, PhD (abd)
Marilyn Frank-Stromborg, RN, EdD, JD, FAAN
Lauri D. John, RN, PhD, CNS
Jan Kinzler, BA
Katen Moore, RN, MSN, ANP-C, AOCN
Giselle J. Moore-Higgs, ARNP, MSN, AOCN
Davina Porock, RN, PhD
Kimberly L. Quinn, RN, MSN, CCRN, CRNP, ACNP
Nancy J. Raymon, RN, MN, AOCN
Paula Trahan Rieger, RN, MSN, CS, AOCN, FAAN
Judy Ross, RN, MSN, ANP-C, AOCN
Dana N. Rutledge, PhD, RN
Diane Spalding, RN, MSN, MBA
Melodie Thomas, RN, BSN, OCN, CCRP
Deborah Lowe Volker, RN, PhD, AOCN
Gail Wilkes, RNC, ANP, MS, AOCN

Also, a special thanks to Judy Phillips, RN, MSN, CCRN, AOCN, FNP-C, for her expertise in chemotherapy and for updating Chapter 8.

PART I

Understanding Lung Cancer

1

Epidemiology and Survival

Trends in Incidence

❖ Lung cancer, referred to as the "unspoken" or ignored cancer, is the most significant public health problem in the United States.

❖ Important changes in the 2003 Cancer statistics—reports are age-adjusted to the United States 2000 population standard rather than 1940s or 1970s database. This new approach results in some dramatic changes in rates of cancer incidence and mortality for different age, racial, and ethnic groups.

❖ Lung cancer is the second most common cancer diagnosed in men and women in the United States; 171,900 estimated new cases of lung cancer were predicted for 2003 (American Cancer Society, 2003a, 2003b).

  ❖ 91,800 new cases in males
  ❖ 80,100 new cases in females

❖ Internationally, lung cancer remains the most common malignancy, with an estimated 1.04 million new cases each year worldwide, accounting for 12.8% of new cancer cases. Fifty-eight percent of new lung cancer cases occur in the developing world. Incidence rates for males is approximately 37.5 new cases per 1 million and 10.8 cases per 1 million for females (Maghfoor, 2002).

❖ Racial differences in the United States: African American males are at least 50% more likely to develop lung cancer than white males. African American females have the highest incidence rates of lung cancer, followed by whites, Asian Pacific Islanders, Hispanics, and American Indians (American Cancer Society, 2001).

❖ Stage of Diagnosis: The majority are diagnosed in late stages for all races (American Cancer Society, 2003b).

  ❖ Localized 15%
  ❖ Regional 24%
  ❖ Distant 48%

❖ 80% of all lung cancers are diagnosed as non-small cell lung cancer (NSCLC).

  ❖ Adenocarcinoma represents 40% of lung cancer cases in the United States, and is the most common form of lung cancer in non-smoking individuals. It is often located peripherally to the bronchi and tends to metastasize to the brain, adrenals, and bone.

- ❖ Squamous cell carcinoma represents 30-35%, mostly occurring centrally near the main stem bronchi, and usually associated with smoking.
- ❖ Large cell carcinoma represents 5-15% and is often located peripherally to bronchi, growing and spreading quickly.

❖ 20% of all lung cancers are diagnosed as small cell lung cancer (SCLC).

- ❖ SCLC tumors tend to be large central masses with extensive mediastinal lymph node metastases; there is also a high likelihood of spreading to distant sites.
- ❖ 95% of SCLC starts in the central part of the chest (ALCASE, 1999).
- ❖ 1/3 of individuals have limited disease, and 2/3 have detectable distant metastases at time of diagnosis (Jeremic et al., 1997; Detterbeck, 2000).

Mortality

❖ Exceeding the combined number of deaths from the second, third, and fourth leading causes of cancer (breast, prostate, and colon cancer, respectively), lung cancer remains the leading cause of death in men and women: 157,200 estimated deaths predicted for 2003 (American Cancer Society, 2003a and 2003b).

- ❖ 88,400 deaths in males
- ❖ 68,800 deaths in females

❖ **Lung and bronchus cancers remain the leading cause of death in older ages.**

  ◆ Males—40-59 years, 60-79 years, and >80 years old
  ◆ Females—60-79 years, >80 years old

❖ Highest mortality rates are for African Americans, followed by whites, American Indian/Alaska Natives, Asian/Pacific Islanders, and Hispanics (respectively).

❖ Internationally, lung cancer is the cause of 921,000 deaths each year, representing 17.8% of cancer-related deaths.

Survival

❖ Primary prognostic factors are histologic cell type and anatomic extent of disease.

❖ Overall, the five-year survival rate for lung cancer in the United States is 15%, compared with 61% for colon cancer, 86% for breast cancer, and 96% for prostate cancer (Alberts, 2003).

❖ Internationally, the survival rates are lower for Europe and the developing world (8%) (BMJ, 2003).

❖ United States racial comparison of five-year relative survival rates at stage of diagnosis (American Cancer Society, 2003):

Staging	*Whites*	*African American*
◆ Localized	49%	43%
◆ Regional	22%	22%
◆ Distant	2%	3%

❖ 5-year survival rate for resectable NSCLC lowers when staged for later disease (Alberg, 2003):

◆ Stage IA	67%
◆ Stage IB	57%
◆ Stage IIA	55%
◆ Stage IIB	39%
◆ Stage IIIA	23%

❖ SCLC individuals with limited stage disease who have undergone chemotherapy and mediastinal irradiation have a median survival of 18-24 months, while those with extensive disease given palliative chemotherapy have a median survival of 10-12 months.

2

Diagnosis, Staging, and Prognosis

Diagnosis Differences

Lung Cancers

❖ Lung cancers are more likely to develop on the right side than on the left (right lung has approximately 55% of the lung parenchyma).

❖ More often than not, upper lobes are involved more than the lower lobes (blood supply to tumors are from bronchial arteries).

❖ Lung cancers can extend the length of the bronchus into the chest wall, across fissures, and into the great vessels, the pericardium, or the diaphragm, and can invade thoracic structures (i.e. superior vena cava), recurrent or phrenic nerves, or esophagus.

❖ Metastases to the mediastinal and pulmonary lymph nodes are common.

❖ Lung cancers can spread to the liver, adrenals, kidneys, brain, and bones.

Small Cell Lung Carcinoma (SCLC)

❖ SCLC is categorized separately because of its rapid proliferation.

❖ SCLC starts in the hormonal cells in the lungs and multiplies rapidly.

❖ Subtypes of SCLC include (see Table 5-1 for histopathological types of lung cancer):
  ❖ Oat cell or lymphocytic
  ❖ Intermediate
  ❖ Combined (small cell combined with squamous or adenocarcinoma)

❖ SCLC is divided into two categories: limited and extensive.

❖ SCLC individuals generally have histories of current or previous smoking, and only 3% of individuals diagnosed with SCLC have no history of active smoking (ALACASE, 1999).

Non-Small Cell Lung Carcinoma (NSCLC)

❖ All subtypes have distinct histologic and clinical characteristics.

❖ Advanced molecular techniques have identified amplification of oncogenes and inactivation of tumor suppressor genes; most important abnormalities are mutations in the *ras* family of oncogenes (ras activation contributes to tumor progression in lung cancer). Of less clear roles in tumor pathogensis and progression are *c-myc* and *c-raf* among oncogenes and retinoblastoma (*Rb*) and *p53* among tumor suppressors (Maghfoor and Perry, 2002).

Lung Cancer Staging for NSCLC Latest Revision[1]—1997

❖ Staging lung cancer is threefold:

  ❖ Allows patients to be grouped on the basis of the disease spread and the expected survival.
  ❖ Appropriate therapy can be applied in a systematic manner once stage is identified.
  ❖ Assists physicians in counseling patients and families regarding potential therapy and prognosis.

❖ Originally adopted in 1986, the staging system for lung cancer began with the International System for Staging Lung Cancer. The last revision was made in 1977 by the American Joint Committee on Cancer (AJCC). AJCC's *Manual for Staging of Cancer* is now considered a universal system for cancer staging to all solid cancers (refer to Tables 5-2 and 5-3 for the latest TNM Staging Classifications, AJCC, 2002).

- ❖ Staging changes:
  - ❖ Stage I tumors were further subdivided into IA and IB. Survival difference based on this distinction has been noted in clinical trial analyses.
  - ❖ Stage II disease was similarly divided into Stage IIA and IIB. Again, A and B were divided to reflect survival differences.
  - ❖ Stage IIIA remains the same except for tumors designated as T3, N0, M0, because the survival of patients with these tumors is similar to that of patients with T2, N1, M0 disease. Consequently, both of these categories are now grouped together as Stage IIB disease.
  - ❖ Stage IIIB and IV remain unchanged except for the changes made to the T4 and M1 descriptors. Specifically, malignant pericardial effusion has been added to the T4 descriptor, the presence of satellite tumors within the lobe of the lung with the primary tumor is classified as T4, and an intrapulmonary ipsilateral distant metastasis is classified as M1.

- ❖ NSCLC can be divided into 3 treatment categories:
  - ❖ Category 1: disease completely contained within the lung and can be completely resected (Stage I and II).
  - ❖ Category 2: tumors that are resectable but are associated with lymph node metastases or

mediastinal involvement that can't be controlled with surgery (Stage IIIA with N2 involvement and Stage IIIB).

* Category 3: tumors associated with distant metastases and given palliative care (Stage IV).

SCLC

❖ TNM staging system does not have the same prognostic significance for individuals with SCLC, and therefore is not utilized.

❖ SCLC is divided into two different categories:

* *Limited* disease (M_0) confined to one side of the chest and nearby lymph nodes. These tumors can generally be encompassed in a tolerable radiation port field for treatment.
* *Extensive* disease (M_1) includes any pleural or pericardial effusion, lung metastases, and massive tumor that would require prohibitive radiation fields (Armstrong, 1998).

Prognosis

❖ For survival rates, refer to earlier discussion and Table 5-4.

❖ Staging is the most important prognostic factor for NSCLC.

- ❖ Early stage disease (Stage I and II) have better prognosis than those who are classified as Stage III and IV.

- ❖ Other factors predicting survival are Karnofsky Performance Scale (KPS) and weight loss.

  - ❖ Low KPS scores correlates with worse outcomes.
  - ❖ Individuals who have loss >5% of body weight during the preceding 3-6 months also have a poor prognosis.

- ❖ Mutations of the *ras* proto-oncogenes, particularly *K-ras*, portend a poor prognosis in individuals with Stage IV NSCLC.

3

Risk Factors

Risk Factors

Background

❖ Lung cancer is one of the few cancers that have identified, specific, known carcinogens.

❖ Focus for healthcare providers should be placed on prevention and reduction to exposure.

❖ American Cancer Society (2003a) estimates 170,000 deaths each year could be avoided if tobacco use were eliminated.

❖ Research continues on diet (fruits, vegetables, and specific antioxidant micronutrients) and its association with lung cancer. Hypotheses suggest diets high in antioxidant nutrients may protect against oxidative DNA damage and thereby protect against lung cancer.

Smoking

❖ Epidemiological studies have convincingly established that nicotine use is the major cause of lung cancer (Armstrong, 1998; Reddy, 2000; Thun et al.,1995).

❖ Smoking is a multi-step carcinogenesis process and causes genetic damage (Mao et al., 1997; Wistuba et al., 1997; Brennan et al., 1995).

❖ 87-90% of all lung cancers are related to smoking (American Cancer Society, 2003a); 78% in males and 90% in females (BMJ, 2003).

❖ Incidence of lung cancer is directly related to the duration of tobacco use and the daily dose of nicotine (Schottenfeld, 1996).

❖ Risk of developing lung cancer for current smokers is 13.3 times higher than those who have never smoked. Risk varies with the number of cigarettes smoked: 10 times over control for those smoking 20 or fewer cigarettes per day to 20 times over control for those smoking more than 20 cigarettes per day (BMJ, 2003).

❖ Second-hand smoke, also referred to as passive smoke, is an indoor carcinogen.

Environmental Factors

❖ Radon, especially for underground miners, was the first occupational respiratory carcinogen, accounting for 10% of lung cancers (Baldwin, Frank, and Fielding, 1998).

❖ Other human occupational agents, accounting for 9-15% of lung cancers, include arsenic, asbestos, chromates, chloromethyl ethers, nickel, polycyclic aromatic hydrocarbons, and radon progeny.

❖ Outdoor air pollutants, accounting for 1-2% of lung cancers, include combustion-generated carcinogens.

❖ Indoor air pollutants: asbestos, radon, cigarette smoke (environmental tobacco smoke), and, in developing countries, cooking stoves and fires.

❖ Unproven but hypothesized are dietary habits, accounting for approximately 20% of lung cancer.

❖ Summary of environmental factors are in Table 5-5 (Alberg and Samet, 2003).

Host Factors

❖ Genetic susceptibility to lung cancer has been postulated, but not yet proven. New techniques of cellular and molecular biology may soon show associations (Alberg and Samet, 2003).

❖ Presence of acquired lung disease:

  ❖ Tuberculosis can develop into lung cancers, particularly in the regions of scar tissue. Risk of lung cancer can be five times greater in men and ten times greater in women who have contracted tuberculosis (Steinitz, 1965). The most common histological type is adenocarcinoma.

* Obstructive airflow (i.e., COPD) or fibrotic disorders restricting lung capacity (pneumoconiosis) remain controversial and have unproven direct associations.

4

Detection and Screening Issues

Introduction

❖ Lung cancer is the number-one killer for males and females, yet no clear guidelines have been established for detection and screening (Ettinger, 2001; American Cancer Society, 2003a, 2003b).

❖ Staging has become very important in detecting lung cancer and determining treatment.

❖ Healthcare providers need to watch for potential warning signs in high-risk patients and follow up with appropriate diagnostic tests.

❖ Health professionals can direct interested individuals to a professionally managed Web site—American Heart and Lung Institute, *http://gek.best.vwh.net*—which provides details on lung cancer screening. This site might aid in patient's understanding and in subsequent discussions with healthcare providers.

❖ Ongoing debates continue concerning the need for and the usefulness of screening for lung cancer (Alberts, 2000; Ettinger, 2001; Jett, 2000; Lee et al., 2001; Reddy, 2000; Bach et.al, 2003).

 ❖ To date, prospective studies of lung cancer screening have not demonstrated persuasively that screening for lung cancer with chest radiography alone or in combination with sputum cytology saves lives. Currently, there are no official recommendations for screening for lung cancer, even in high-risk populations.

 ❖ Readers should recognize that this area is rapidly changing, and screening should be based on shared, informed decision making between the healthcare provider and the patient.

❖ Current technologies that aid in detecting early-stage lung cancer are presented and evaluated in this section. It is imperative that every healthcare professional understand the specificity and sensitivity of each test and the advantages and disadvantages to each diagnostic test.

Diagnostic Test: Chest X-ray

❖ Chest radiography is probably one of the most valuable tools in the diagnoses of lung cancer.

❖ Sensitivity of chest X-ray for lung cancer detection is dependent on:

 1. Size and location of the lesion

2. Quality assurance factors related to image quality

3. Skill of the interpreting physician (Ginsberg, Vokes, and Rosenzweig, 2001; Armstrong, 1998)

❖ Failure to detect lesions at a favorable size, or even at a larger size, can occur because the mediastinum, ribs, and other aspects of chest structure may obstruct them. Errors in perception on the part of the interpreter are also common.

❖ Early 1980s utilizing annual chest X-rays in screening trials didn't show any reductions in lung cancer mortality. Trials were not sensitive at detecting lesions < 2 cm in size, and patients with chronic obstructive pulmonary disease had a four- to six-fold increased risk of lung cancer independent of their smoking history (Jett, 2000).

❖ The Prostate, Lung, Colorectal, and Ovarian (PLCO) Cancer Screening Trial started recruitment in 1994, and initial findings are that serial chest x-rays shows no proven benefits for individuals without symptoms or history of cancer (Prorok et.al., 2000).

Sputum Cytology

❖ Sputum cytology, believed to have potential for early detection of lung cancer, didn't show added advantage over chest X-ray in the National Cancer Institute (NCI) cooperative trials; it was also not associated with any reduction in deaths from lung cancer (Berlin et al., 1984). In those trials, approximately one in four cancers were detected by sputum cytology alone, and the majority of these were squamous cell carcinomas diagnosed at a favorable stage. Although sputum cytology is the least invasive means of obtaining a specific diagnosis in a patient suspected of having lung cancer, this method is not necessarily the easiest to perform; it is very dependent on rigorous specimen sampling and preservation techniques. Average overall sensitivity is 64% but it drops lower for peripheral lesions of 40% (Detterbeck, 2000).

❖ Attempts to refine the use of sputum cytology, however, are continuing. Earlier randomized, controlled studies in the United States tested whether a combination of chest X-rays and sputum examination could be more effective than either alone or by utilizing practice guidelines in detecting early lung cancer (persistent cough, shortness of breath, hoarseness, hemoptyosis, and so on). Studies found that prospective screening practice guideline programs for lung cancer did not have any significant improvement in overall survival rates compared with using chest X-rays and sputum cytology (Minna et al., 1997).

❖ Review of 5 randomized clinical trials (London 1960-1964, Mayo 1971-1983, Czechoslovakia

1976-1980, MSKCC 1974-1982, and Johns
Hopkins 1973-1982) suggest neither chest X-ray
or sputum cytology are proven screening tests
(Bach, Kelley, Tae, and McCrory, 2003).

Low-Radiation-Dose Computed Tomography (Spiral or Helical CT)

❖ Low-radiation spiral computed tomography (CT)
  is a diagnostic test scanning the entire chest in 15
  seconds while holding a single breath, and provides 5 mm multiplanar slices of the chest. It is
  more sensitive than chest X-ray in the detection
  of small pulmonary nodules, mediastinum
  adenopathy, small pleural effusions, and the ability to detect abnormalities below the diaphragm
  (Schoepf, 2001).

❖ Introduction of CT scanning in the late 1970s was
  a giant step forward and probably the most promising new tool for early lung cancer screening.

❖ CT has the potential to detect 75–80% of lung
  cancers in Stage I (Jett, 2000). The Early Lung
  Cancer Project (ELCAP), which is still ongoing, is
  a nonrandomized trial designed to evaluate
  screening with low-radiation-dose CT. In a baseline report (Henschke et al., 1999, 2001) with
  1,000 volunteers aged 60 years and older with a
  smoking history of at least ten pack-years, and
  who would be acceptable candidates for thoracic

surgery, low-dose CT significantly outperformed conventional chest X-ray in the detection of small pulmonary nodules. Noncalcified pulmonary nodules were detected three times as commonly (23% vs 7%), malignancies four times as commonly (2.7% vs 0.7%) and Stage I malignancies six times as commonly (2.3% vs 0.4%).

❖ Still, the debate continues as to whether spiral CT is a beneficial screening test that can meet two criteria (Bach, Kelley, Tate, and McCrory, 2003):

   ❖ Screening test must provide benefit to individuals who have the illness by increasing life expectancy

   ❖ Screening test should not be dangerous or painful and should not have numerous false-positive results that cause anxiety or necessitate invasive follow-up tests

Positron Emission Tomography (PET)

❖ Positron emission tomography (PET) scanning is a relatively new technology. Discriminating between cells that are rapidly dividing, PET scans detect tumor physiology as opposed to anatomy. They are thought to be potentially more sensitive than CT scans (Patz and Erasmus, 1999; Gould et al., 2001).

❖ Studies have reported PET scans' mediastinal node sampling sensitivity is 88% and average specificity is 94% (Detterbeck, 2000). This is probably why there has been more interest in using

PET scanning, especially to evaluate mediastinal nodes, since CT scanning has known limitations for evaluating these lymph nodes.

❖ Even though the sensitivity and specificity of PET scanning is high, limitations are:

❖ Poor anatomic location of the tumor—sometimes it is difficult to differentiate hilar nodes from mediastinal nodes

❖ High cost

❖ Limited availability

❖ False readings—false positives can occur with infectious and inflammatory lesions and false negatives may occur with tumors of low metabolic activity, small tumors, and in hyperglycemic states. A recent comparison study evaluated by Pieterman and colleagues (2000) between the sensitivity and specificity of CT versus PET for the detection of mediastinal metastases in patients with NSCLC showed higher rates for PET scanning. (PET sensitivity 91% and specificity 86% as compared to CT, which was 75% and 66%, respectively.)

❖ The National Comprehensive Cancer Network (NCCN), which has written numerous cancer guidelines, does not yet recommend PET scanning as part of the routine initial evaluation of NSCLC (Demetri et al., 1996). NCCN does recognize the promising value it can add in pretreatment and post-treatment to follow up chest

X-rays, CT, or MRI scans. Although PET scanning
may not yet be recognized as the standard, excit-
ing information was released at the 36th Annual
Meeting of the American Society of Clinical
Oncology (2001): PET scans predict survival and
prevent unnecessary surgery in NSCLC. An
Australian physician, Dr. MacManus (2000),
found correlations between favorable PET scan
results and survival rates. Also, Dutch researchers
from nine institutions found PET scans were very
accurate and indeed prevented futile thoraco-
tomies (MacManus, 2000).

❖ Although Medicare does not set standards, it has
expanded its coverage for PET scans. Effective
July 1, 2001, PET scans are covered for diagnosis, initial staging, and restaging of NSCLC
(Medicare Bulletin, 2001). The Medicare Bulletin
also contains further explanation as to whether
PET scans are to be used for staging and/or
restaging when the stage of cancer is "in doubt"
after a standard diagnostic workup is completed
by CT or MRI.

Magnetic Resonance Imaging (MRI)

❖ MRI investigation of pulmonary lesions has been
disappointing and has offered no improvement
over CT scanning, except to evaluate the extent of
tumor invasion or destruction of peripheral structures such as the brachial plexus, vertebral body,

and spinal canal. MRIs may be of value in clinical Stage III disease if combined-modality therapy is being considered (Scott, 2000).

Bronchoscopies

❖ Image-guided transthoracic bronchoscopy's fine-needle aspirations (FNA) have revolutionized lung cancer staging. This procedure facilitates precise biopsy of lung lesions and virtually all mediastinal lymph node areas (Harrow et al., 2000; Savage and Zwischenberger, 2000). Because chest X-rays, CT, and PET scanning identify suspicious lesions only, they cannot make a tissue differential. Transthoracic bronchoscopies have allowed for less invasive and costly diagnostic testing offering high yields.

❖ In 1996, the FDA approved an even newer device known as autoflourescence bronchoscopy (Xillix LIFE-Lung), allowing physicians to observe whether cells fluoresce or reflect light normally. Fluorescent dye is injected into and taken up by the tumor cells; the dye causes the cells to fluoresce under blue light. If the cells do not fluoresce normally, a sample is taken to determine whether they are cancerous. This technique is used in special circumstances when ordinary bronchoscopy fails to reveal a tumor detected by sputum cytology. One multicentered trial reported a higher sensitivity (2.7 times) in detecting carcinomas utilizing LIFE bronchoscopies as compared to the normal use of white light bronchoscopies (Jett, 2000).

Genetic Markers

❖ Researchers are investigating genetic markers or "fingerprints" to detect the presence of cancer cells. These markers are found in blood samples utilizing highly sophisticated laboratory tests. Unfortunately, no genetic markers are available yet to detect and diagnose early-stage lung cancer (AJCC, 2002).

❖ Recently, there has been excitement and emphasis on the identification of the p53 tumor suppressor gene. Scientists have been investigating the p53 tumor suppressor gene, which influences DNA repair and cell death, in both NSCLC and SCLC. P53 slows down DNA destruction. Studies are being conducted to inject normal p53 genes into tumors, thus deterring cancer growth.

5

Key Clinical Implications for Understanding Lung Cancer

Key Clinical Points

❖ Diagnosis of lung cancer depends on identifying the "type" of lung cancer (NSCLC or SCLC), size and location of primary tumor, presence or absence of metastases, and overall clinical status of patient.

❖ 80% of all lung cancers are diagnosed as NSCLC; 20% are SCLC.

❖ SCLC is more aggressive than NSCLC and is often extensive-stage at time of diagnosis.

❖ Early stage NSCLC (Stage I and II) have better prognosis and outcomes than later stage (Stage III and IV).

❖ Clinical staging determines treatment options; diagnostic tests include chest X-ray, CT scans, PET scans, and MRI.

❖ Sputum cytology, chest radiography, and fiber-optic bronchoscopy have shown only limited effectiveness in lung cancer screening.

❖ Important prognostic factors are histologic cell type and disease spread (liver, adrenals, kidneys, brain, and bones).

❖ Risk factors, some which are preventable, include smoking, and radon exposure, along with other pollutants, and genetics though not totally conclusive.

❖ Lung cancer is number one killer for males and females in U.S.

TABLE 5-1
Histopathologic Types of Malignant Epithelial Tumors, World Health Organization

Small Cell Carcinoma	Adenocarcinoma	Large Cell Carcinoma
Oat cell carcinoma	Acinar adenocarcinoma	Giant cell carcinoma variant
Intermediate cell type	Papillary adenocarcinoma	Clear cell carcinoma variant
Combined oat cell carcinoma	Bronchiolo-alveolar carcinoma	
	Solid carcinoma with mucus formation	

Squamous cell carcinoma (epidermoid)
Spindle cell variant

Adenosquamous Carcinoma	Carcinoid

Bronchial gland carcinoma	Others
Adenoid cystic carcinoma	
Mucoepidermoid carcinoma	

Yesner et al. 1997

TABLE 5–2 AJCC STAGING OF LUNG CANCER

Primary Tumor (T)

TX	Primary tumor cannot be assessed, or tumor proven by presence of malignant cells in sputum or bronchial washings but cannot be visualized by imaging or bronchoscopy
T0	No evidence of primary tumor
T*is*	Carcinoma *in situ*
T1	Tumor 3 cm or less in greatest dimension, surrounded by lung or visceral pleura, without bronchoscopic evidence of invasion more proximal than the lobar bronchus (i.e., not in main bronchus)
T2	Tumor with any of the following features of size or extent:
	More than 3 cm in greatest dimension
	Involves main bronchus, 2 cm or more distal to the carina
	Invades the visceral pleura
	Associated with atelectasis or obstructive pneumonitis that extends to the hilar region but does not involve the entire lung
T3	Tumor of any size that directly invades any of the following: chest wall (including superior sulcus tumors), diaphragm, mediastinal pleura, parietal pericardium; or tumor in the main bronchus less than 2 cm distal to the carina but without involvement of the carina; or associated atelectasis of obstructive pneumonitis of the entire lung
T4	Tumor of any size that invades any of the following: mediastinum, heart, great vessels, trachea, esophagus, vertebral body, carina; separate tumor nodule(s) in the same lobe; or tumor with a malignant pleural effusion

Regional Lymph Nodes (N)

NX	Regional lymph nodes cannot be assessed
N0	No regional lymph node metastasis
N1	Metastasis to ipsilateral peribronchial and/or ipsilateral hilar lymph nodes and intrapulmonary nodes involved by direct extension of the primary tumor
N2	Metastasis to ipsilateral mediastinal and/or subcarinal lymph node(s)
N3	Metastasis in contralateral mediastinal, contralateral hilar, ipsilateral or contralateral scalene or supraclavicular lymph node(s)

Distant Metastasis (M)

MX	Distant metastasis cannot be assessed
M0	No distant metastasis
M1	Distant metastasis present (includes synchronous separate nodule(s) in a different lobe)

TABLE 5-3
Stage Grouping

Stage grouping of the TNM subsets has been revised as follows. TNM refers to primary tumor (T), regional lymph node (N), and distant metastasis (M).

Occult Carcinoma	TX	N0	M0
Stage 0	T*is*	N0	M0
Stage IA	T1	N0	M0
Stage IB	T2	N0	M0
Stage IIA	T1	N1	M0
Stage IIB	T2	N1	M0
	T3	N0	M0
Stage IIIA	T1	N2	M0
	T2	N2	M0
	T3	N1	M0
	T3	N2	M0
Stage IIIB	Any T	N3	M0
	T4	Any N	M0
Stage IV	Any T	Any N	M1

Used with the permission of the American Joint Committee on Cancer (AJCC), Chicago, Illinois. The original source for this material is the *AJCC Cancer Staging Manual, Sixth Edition* (2002) published by Springer-Verlag New York, www.springer-ny.com.

TABLE 5-4
Overall Survival of NSCLC: Clinically Staged Versus Pathologically Staged*

	Overall Survival Clinically Staged	*Overall Survival Pathologically Staged*
T1N0	67%	73%
T2N0	41%	62%

T1N1	34%	61%
T2N1	26%	42%
T3N0	27%	40%

Mountain, 1997

*Clinical staging is based on minimally invasive tests and pathologic staging is based on operative findings

TABLE 5-5
Environmental Pollutants Associated with Lung Cancer

Asbestos exposure

Aluminum production

Arsenic exposure

Cadmium exposure

Chloromethyl ethers

Chromium exposure

Coal gasification

Coke production

Household combustion devices

Nickel

Radon gas

Soot exposure

Tobacco smoke (first/second-hand)

Uranium exposure

Alberg and Samet, 2003

References: Chapters 1–5

Alberg, A. and Samet, J. (2003). Epidemiology of lung cancer. *Chest*, 123(1): 21–49.

ALCASE. (1999). *The Lung Cancer Manual.* Vancouver, Washington: Alliance for Lung Cancer Advocacy.

American Cancer Society. (2001). *Cancer Facts and Figures.* New York: American Cancer Society.

American Cancer Society. (2003). Cancer statistics, 2003. *CA: A Cancer Journal for Clinicans.* 53(l): Lippincott Williams and Wilkins.

American Cancer Society. (2003). *Cancer Facts and Figures.* New York: American Cancer Society.

American Cancer Society. (2001). *Cancer Facts and Figures for African Americans 2000-2001.* New York: American Cancer Society.

American Joint Committee on Cancer. (2002). *AJCC Cancer Staging Manual.* 6th ed., Philadelphia: Lippincott-Raven.

Armstrong, J. (1998). Tumors of the lung and mediastium. In: Leibel, S., Phillips, T. (eds.). *Textbook of Radiation Oncology.* Philadelphia: WB Saunders Company.

Bach, Kelley, Tae, and McCrory. (2003). Screening for Lung Cancer: A Review of the Current Literature. *Chest* volume 123, Number 1. 2003 Supplement pg 72–82

Baldwin, G., Frank, E., and Fielding, B. (1998). U.S. Women physicians' residential radon testing practices. *American Journal of Preventive Medicine,* 15(1), 49–53.

Berlin, N., Buncher, C., Fontana, R., Frost, J., and Melaned, M. (1984). The National Cancer Institute Cooperative Early Lung Cancer Detection Program. *American Reference Respiratory Disease,* 130(4): 545–549.

Bonner, J. (2000). Non-small cell lung cancer. *Seminars in Radiation Oncology,* 10(4) October: 263–266.

BMJ. (2003). *Clinical Evidence Concise: The International Source of the Best Available Evidence for Effective Health Care.* G. Jones (editor). London, UK. BMJ Publishing Company.

Brennan, J., Boyle, J., Koch, W., et al. (1995). Association between cigarette smoking and mutation of the p53 gene in squamous-cell carcinoma of the head and neck. *New England Journal of Medicine,* 332(11): 712–717.

Brown, J. (2000). Non-small cell lung cancer. *Seminars in Radiation Oncology.* 10(4): 263–266.

CARMA. (2000). *How the media report on cancer: An analysis of lung, breast, colorectal and prostate cancer coverage: October Report.* Washington, DC: Computer Aided Research and Media Analysis International, USA.

Demetri, G., Elias, A., Gersheason, D., Fossella, F., Grecula, J., Mittal, B. (1996). NCCN small cell lung cancer practice guidelines. The national comprehensive cancer network. *Oncology,* 11(10) November: 179–94.

Detterbeck, F. (2000). Diagnosis and staging of non-small cell lung cancer. Diagnosis and treatment of lung cancer: An evidence-based guide for the practicing clinician. *Chest,* 1(2): 1–13.

Ettinger, D. (2001). New NCCN recommendations for non-small cell lung cancer. *Oncology News International,* 10(4): 1, 39.

Ginsberg, R., Kris, M., and Armstrong, J. (1993). Non-small cell lung cancer. In: De Vita, V.T., Hellman, S., Rosenberg, S. (eds.). *Principles and Practice of Oncology.* Philadelphia: JB Lippincott.

Ginsberg, R., Vokes, E., and Rosenzweig, K. (2001). *Non-Small Cell Lung Cancer. Principles and Practice of Oncology.* 6th ed., Philadelphia: Lippincott Williams and Wilkins.

Gould, M., Maclean, C., Kuschner, W., Rydzak, C., and Owens, D. (2001). Accuracy of positron emission tomography for diagnosis of pulmonary nodules and mass lesions. *Journal of the American Medical Association,* 285(7): 914–924.

Harrow, E., Abi-Salch, W., Blum J., Harkin, T., Gasparini, S., Addrizzo, B., Arroliga, A., Wight, G., and Mehta, A. (2000). The utility of transbronchial needle aspiration in the staging of bronchogenic carcinoma. *American Journal of Respiratory Critical Care Medicine,* 161: 601–607.

Henschke, C., McCauley, D., Yankelevitz, D., Naidich, D., McGuinnes, G., Olli, S., Miettinen, O., Libby, D., Pasmantier, M., Kolzumi, J., Altorki, N., and Smith, I. (1999). Is quality of life predictive of the survival of patients with advanced non-small cell lung cancer? *Cancer,* 8(2), 333–340.

Henschke, C., McCauley, D., Yankelevitz, D., Naidich, D., McGuinnes, G., Olli, S., Miettinen, O., Libby, D., Pasmantier, M., Kolzumi, J., Altorki, N., and Smith, I. (2001). Early Lung Cancer Action Project: A summary of the findings on baseline screening. *The Oncologist,* 6: 147–152.

Jeremic, B., Shibamoto, Y., Acimovic, L., and Milisavljevic, S. (1997). Initial versus delayed accelerated hyperfactionated radiation therapy and concurrent chemotherapy in limited small cell lung cancer: A randomized study. *International Journal of Radiation Oncology Biology and Physics,* 50(1): 19–25.

Maghfoor, I. and Perry, M. (2002). Lung cancer, non-small cell. http://www.emedicine.com/med/topic 1333.htm

Mao, L., Lee, J., Kurie, J., Fan Y., Lippman, S., Lee, J., Ro, J., Jroxson, A., Yu, R., Morice, R., Kemp, B., Khuri, F., Walsh, G., Hittelman, W., and Hong, W. (1997). Clonal genetic alterations in the lungs of current and former smokers. *Journal of the National Cancer Institute,* 89(12): 857–862.

Martini, N. (1995). Mediastinal lymph node dissection for lung cancer. *Chest Surgery Clinical North America:* 189–203.

Mountain, R. (1997). Revisions in the international system for staging lung cancer. *Chest,* 11: 1710–1717.

Patz, E. and Eramus, J. (1999). Positron emission tomography imaging in lung cancer. *Clinical Lung Cancer,* 1: 42–28.

Pieterman, R., van Putten, J., Meuzelaar, J., Mooyaart, E., Vaalburg, W., Koeter, G., Pruim, J., and Groen, H. (2000). Preoperative staging of non-small cell lung cancer with positron-emission tomography. *New England Journal of Medicine,* 343: 254–261.

Prorok, P., Andriole, G., Bresalier, R., et. al (2000). Design of the Prostate, Lung, Colorectal and Ovarian (PLCO) Cancer Screening Trial. *Control Clinical Trials.* 21(6 suppl): 2735-3095.

Reddy, A. (2000). *Non-Small Cell Lung Cancer: Imaging and Staging.* American Society for Therapeutic Radiology and Oncology, 42nd Annual Meeting, October 22, 2000.

Savage, C. and Zwischenberger, J. (2000). Image-guided fine needle aspirate strategies for staging of lung cancer. *Clinical Lung Cancer,* 2(2): 101–110.

Schoepf, J. (2001). Lung cancer screening with 1mm multi-slice CT scans. *Oncology News International,* 10(1): 10.

Schottenfield, D. (1996). Epidemiology of Lung Cancer. In: Pass, H., Mitchell, J., Johnson, D., and Turrisi, A. (eds.). *Lung Cancer: Principles and Practice.* New York: Lippincott-Raven.

Scott, W. (2000). *Lung Cancer: A Guide to Diagnosis and Treatment.* Omaha, Nebraska: Atticas Books.

Steinitz, R. (1965). Pulmonary tuberculosis and carcinoma of the lung: A survey from two population-based disease registers. *American Respiratory Diseases,* 92: 758–766.

Thun, M., Day-Lally, C., Calle, E., Flanders, W., and Heath, C. (1995). Excess mortality among cigarette smokers: Changes in a 20-year-interval. *American Journal of Public Health,* 85: 1223–1230.

Wistuba, I., Lam S., Behrens, C., Virmani, A., Fong, K., LeRiche, J., Srivastava, S., Minna, J., and Gazdar, F. (1997). Molecular damage in the bronchial epithelium of current and former smokers. *Journal of the National Cancer Institute,* 889(18): 1366–1373.

Yesner, R., Sobin, L., et al. (1997). *Histologic Typing of Lung Tumors, Revised.* Geneva: World Health Organization.

PART II

Standard Treatment Modalities

6

Pretreatment Evaluation

Work-Up

❖ At presentation, >90% of patients with lung cancer will be symptomatic (Tan, Flaherty, Kazerooni, and Iannettoni, 2003).

❖ Initial History and Physical Examination includes:

  ❖ Symptoms if suspect primary lung tumor:

    ❖ Cough (most common presenting symptom)
    ❖ Dyspnea (develops in 60% of individuals, tumor may block airway causing breathlessness) along with wheezing and stridor
    ❖ Hemoptysis (common, rarely severe, usually consists of blood streaked sputum)
    ❖ Chest discomfort (occurs up to 50% of individuals, usually described as intermittent and aching in quality, very ill-defined in nature, if spread to the pleural surface will complain of pleuritic chest pain)

- ❖ Symptoms if suspect intrathoracic spread:
  - ❖ Recurrent laryngeal nerve palsy (occurs in 2-18%, more common in left-sided tumors because of the laryngeal nerve around the aortic arch, causes hoarseness)
  - ❖ Phrenic nerve dysfunction (evident by elevated hemidiaphragm on chest X-ray)
  - ❖ Horner's syndrome: invasion of the sympathetic ganglion by an apical lung tumor causing ptosis, enophthalmos, small pupil on one side of the face, and ipsilateral anhydrosis
  - ❖ Superior vena cava (SVC) syndrome: complaints of facial swelling, including neck and eyelids, with dilated veins on upper chest, shoulders, and arms. Also can cause dizziness (especially bending or leaning forward), drowsiness, blurred vision, cough, and dysphagia
- ❖ Thoracic symptoms: cough, shortness of breath, dyspnea, hemoptyosis
- ❖ Adenopathy: cervical and supraclavicular lymph nodes; (enlargement of lymph nodes may be the first clue of nodal metastasis (N3 disease), which will dictate treatment (chemotherapy, radiation therapy or both)
- ❖ Karnofsky Performance Status: KPS scores, evaluation of cardiac function, pulmonary function, exercise tolerance
- ❖ Co-morbid conditions: COPD (influencing therapy options)

* Weight loss: usually more than 10% of body weight

❖ Diagnostic Tests—complete workup is required to assess tumor and possible metastasis dissemination. Common sites of distant metastasis from lung cancer are: bones, liver, adrenal glands, intra-abdominal lymph nodes, brain/spinal cord, lymph nodes, and skin (Beckles, Spiro, Colice, and Rudd, 2003a). Available tests include:

  * **Blood analyses:** complete blood counts and metabolic profiles are standard tests to evaluate various organ function
  * **Chest radiography:** provides information on the size, shape, and density of the tumor; indicates presence of thoracic lymphadenopathy, pleural effusion, pericardial effusion, pulmonary infiltrates, pneumonia, and/or consolidation. Also, bone metastases can be visualized.
  * **Pulmonary function tests:** important predictors of a person's ability to undergo surgical resection or withstand irradiation
  * **Bone scan:** warranted when patients complain of persistent bone pain in trunk or extremities
  * **MRI:** evaluate suspected spinal cord compression, or, if SCLC is suspected, a brain MRI/CT is justified
  * **CT of chest and upper abdomen (including the adrenals):** details more about the tumor's surface characteristics, enlargement of lymph

nodes, location, and position in regards to the mediastinum and mediastinal structures, metastasis to lung, bones, liver, and adrenals

❖ **Bronchoscopy:** biopsy is required to determine whether the nodes are involved with lung cancer metastasis and the extent of spread

  ❖ Transbronchial biopsy: passing a special 21-gauge needle through the flexible bronchoscope to biopsy mediastinal nodes or other masses adjacent to the large bronchi

  ❖ Fluorescence bronchoscopy: IV injection of hematoporphyrin derivatives that localize in situ and superficial tumors as they fluoresce when illuminated with light

❖ **Endoscopic ultrasound:** aids in staging the mediastinum metastases

❖ **Video-assisted thoracic surgery:** used to biopsy left hilar lymph nodes and evaluate the intrathoracic manifestations of the lung tumor

❖ **Transthoracic needle aspiration biopsy:** fine-needle aspiration (FNA) by transthoracic route is another option for those patients who are unable to undergo surgery

❖ **Positron emission tomography (PET):** cancer cells metabolize glucose (fluorodeoxyglucose or FDG) more rapidly than normal cells, thus being visualized on the nuclear scan. Can indicate whether tumor is growing or shrinking over different time intervals but typically cannot pinpoint exact location

❖ **Combined PET/CT Scanner:** integrated PET-CT scans have better diagnostic accuracy than other CT or PET alone. Tumor and nodal staging has been found to be significantly more accurate (Lardinois et. al, 2003). Therefore, integrated PET-CT can improve the ability to diagnose lung cancer, determine how far it has spread, and track patients' responses to treatment.

❖ **Molecular marker assays:** currently under investigation to detect lung cancer in its earliest stages

  ❖ DNA aneuploidy is associated with poor survival
  ❖ Ki-67 is a predictor of distant metastases
  ❖ Oncogene (k-ras, myc, neu) mutations in these genes are found in lung cancers and associated with poor survival
  ❖ Tumor suppressor genes such as p-53, and retinoblastoma (RB) also predict poor survival

7

Surgical Treatment and Other Invasive Therapeutic Options

Introduction

❖ Anatomic resection of lung cancer is the gold standard for treatment of early-stage NSCLC (Stage I, II, or even early IIIA). However, since SCLC presents in advance stages, surgery is typically not an option.

❖ Pre-operative physiologic assessment for surgical resection should consider: immediate perioperative risks from comorbid cardiopulmonary disease, long-term risks of pulmonary disability, and the threat to survival due to reoccurrence (Beckles, Spiro, Colice, and Rudd, 2003b).

❖ Improved smaller resections over the years have led to lower mortality rates. These include sleeve resection, bronchoplastic procedures, segmentectomy, and lobectomy.

❖ With the introduction of surgical staplers, lung resections are now safer, faster, and less traumatic to patients.

❖ Other therapeutic treatment modalities are available for endobronchial malignancies: photodynamic therapy (PDT), electrocautery, cryotherapy, and Nd-YAG laser therapy. Brachytherapy is also available and is presented in Chapter 9.

Goal of Surgical Therapy

❖ The goal of surgical therapy is complete resection of the lung cancer, while preserving the remaining lung, where cure is the ultimate aim.

❖ Surgical considerations are:

  ❖ Patient must first be deemed resectable and operable prior to surgery. A resectable patient is one who has disease that is still local or locoregional in scope, which can be removed with surgery (Johnston, 1997).

  ❖ Every NSCLC patient with locoregional should be approached as a potential candidate for resection (LoCicero, Ponn, and Daly, 2000).

  ❖ Age alone should not be a deterrent from offering thoracic surgery. The mortality rate of the elderly (>70 years old) for lobectomies is between 4-7%, and for pneumonectomies, 14% (Beckles, Spiro, Colice, and Rudd, 2003a). Critical assessment should be based on physical condition and other co-morbidities (cardiac disease, diabetes, and chronic obstructive pulmonary disease) rather than strictly age.

❖ Patients presenting with malignant pleural effusions have increased risk of microvascular permeability, thus surgery may not be an option. The patient may require other medical-oncological therapy, such as chemotherapy and radiation therapy.

❖ Clinical trials have shown no survival benefit with pre-operative radiation therapy as compared to surgery alone (Komaki, 1985; Komaki et al, 1985). Likewise, post-operative radiation has no significant survival benefit in patients without evidence of lymphatic metastasis (Weisenburger, 1994).

❖ Criteria for surgical resections:

1. Establishment or confirmation of the diagnosis; this is done by radiographic studies and biopsies, specifically chest X-rays, chest CT scans, and biopsies
2. Complete resection of the tumor is possible
3. Systematic sampling or complete dissection of lymph nodes draining to the primary tumor is performed (achieved by a pulmonary resection, but can be done by mediastinoscopy)

Diagnostic Assessment

❖ Radiographic studies would include a computed

tomography (CT) scan of the thorax, or possibly a positron emission tomography (PET) scan.

* CT scan is utilized to evaluate solitary pulmonary nodules. CT scans of the thorax rely on the fact that malignant tumors are highly vascularized and therefore are enhanced by intravenous contrast material (Reed and Silvestri, 2000)
* PET scans preoperative are controversial. PET scans help to evaluate indeterminate pulmonary lesions, but it can present with false positives. Sometimes these false positives can be the result of active infectious or inflammatory lesions (Reed and Silvestri, 2000). Also, false negatives can occur with low metabolic activity. Carcinoid tumors are a type of malignancy that may yield a false negative result. PET scans helps the thoracic surgeon in recommending further invasive testing or resection options.

* Invasive assessments include either a fine-needle biopsy, bronchoscopy, and/or mediastinoscopy.

    * **Fine-needle biopsy:** procedure of choice for the diagnosis of peripheral pulmonary nodules. Salazar and Wescott (1993) reported accuracy of between 80–90%.
    * **Bronchoscopy:** can diagnose, stage, and in some cases, treat lung cancer. It is the procedure of choice in patients with centrally located masses. The diagnostic yield of

fiberoptic bronchosocopy for centrally located lung masses presumed to be cancer is approximately 70% and increases to greater than 90% when the lesion is visualized in the airway (Reed and Silvestri, 2000).

* **Mediastinoscopy:** a common, safe procedure used for the diagnosis of thoracic disease and staging of lung cancer (Hammound et al., 1999). Mediastinoscopy can be a very controversial procedure and some would argue that it is unnecessary, especially if the patient will undergo pulmonary resection. Resection may take place despite the results of the mediastinoscopy. In patients with Stage III and Stage IV disease, a mediastinoscopy will provide the necessary information to help plan the necessary adjuvant therapy.

Operative Criteria for Surgical Resection

* Patient's suitability for thoracic surgery includes:

  * **Mental preparedness:** assess patients' willingness to seek treatment or their anxiety with their lung cancer. If focusing on their disease and the potential for a poor outcome, it can lead to depression. Depression is common in the cancer patient and left untreated, may lead to a poor surgical outcome. Medications are available that can help combat some of the symptoms that a depressed patient may be

experiencing. Conversely, a positive attitude enhances how a patient feels about the potential prognosis and disease process.

* **Physiological health:** strong cardiac and pulmonary status are essential. Lung resection decreases the pulmonary vascular bed and can result in an acute increase in right ventricular and pulmonary artery pressure leading to right ventricular failure. Decreased lung compliance and diffusion capacity, with a resultant increase in the work of breathing, may aggravate a pre-existing cardiac disease or lead to new onset ischemia.

  * Although cardiac morbidity is rare, those patients that suffered a myocardial infarction just three months prior to having surgery have an increased risk of surgical mortality. The risk of perioperative infarction is inversely related to the time interval between the original myocardial infarction and the surgical procedure (Alexander and Anderson, 2000). This relationship follows a curvilinear, rather than linear, relationship.

  * The effect of pulmonary parenchymal resection on postoperative pulmonary function should be a consideration. All patients being considered for thoracotomy should have pulmonary function tests (PFTs) performed to assess a patients' pulmonary reserve (Reilly, 1999). Specifically, the forced vital capacity

(FEV1) and the diffusion lung capacity (DLCO) are assessed.

- ❖ The FEV1 measures a patient's forced expiratory volume. Patients that are considered high risk are those with an FEV1 less than 0.7 L and/or 40% predicted.
- ❖ The DLCO measures carbon monoxide and reflects the efficiency of gas exchange (Reilly, 1999). A patient's DLCO should measure greater than 60% predicted. Any patient receiving any values less than those mentioned here should not receive surgery until further workup is performed by a pulmonologist.

Thoracic Incisions

- ❖ For many years the posterolateral thoracotomy was considered the incision of choice for most operations involving the esophagus and lung.

- ❖ With increased use of double-lumen endotracheal tubes and refinement of instrumentation, especially stapling techniques, the posterolateral thoracotomy is reserved for the more difficult case (Fry, 2000).

- ❖ Today, the most popular incision for open general thoracic surgical procedures is the lateral thoracotomy, (referred to as the axillary thoracotomy).

- ❖ Surgical differences:

❖ A **posterolateral thoracotomy** incision is made with the patient in a left lateral decubitus position with padding to the elbows, knees, and dependent axilla. The "S" shaped incision starts in front of the anterior axillary line, curves 4 cm under the tip of the scapula, and takes a vertical direction between the posterior midline over the vertebral column and medial edge of the scapula. Rib resection is recommended for patients over 40 years of age to decrease the incidence of rib fracture. The main advantage to this technique is the superb exposure for most thoracic procedures. The disadvantage is the length of the incision and amount of muscle and soft tissue transected.

❖ **Lateral thoracotomy,** originally developed for operations on the upper thoracic sympathetic nerve system, is useful when a double-lumen endotracheal tube is used, as in an uncomplicated pulmonary resection. Additionally, the only muscle transected with this incision is the intercostal muscle group. The chief advantages of this incision are the speed of opening and closing, the reduced blood loss from minimal muscle transection, and the resulting reduced postoperative discomfort (Fry, 2000). In preparation for the procedure, the patient is positioned in a lateral decubitus position with the arm abducted at 90 degrees and positioned on an armrest. A sequential compression device is applied on the legs and an axillary roll is placed. Due to the limited exposure of the axillary thoracotomy incision, it should only be performed by an experienced thoracic surgeon. It is a useful incision that deserves wider application than it has received, and it is associated with less postoperative discomfort than a posterolateral thoracotomy or median sternotomy (Fry, 2000).

Operative Procedures

❖ Two key factors when deciding the type of thoracic surgery are tumor location and the surgical experience of the surgeon.

❖ Common types of thoracic surgery performed are lobectomy, pulmonary wedge resection, sleeve resection, and pneumonectomy:

   ❖ **Lobecotomy:** a standard surgical resection for Stage I tumors performed when cancer is confined to a single lobe, along with associated pleural and drainage pathways (Shields, 2000). Due to high success rates, adjuvant therapy is typically not done outside clinical trials. Several studies are now being done to determine whether chemotherapy administered before or after surgery is beneficial in reducing the number of recurrences. 5-year survival rates on recurrence is significant for T1N0M0 patients at 80%, and at 85% for patients with T2N0M0 lesions (Martini et al., 1999). The benefit of adjuvant therapy in this population is dually dependent on the availability of effective therapies and methods to follow patients for response or failure (Harwood, 1996). To date, no additional adjuvant therapy is recommended. More information can be found at *www.your-surgery.com,* by selecting Chest and then Thoracotomy.

❖ **Pulmonary wedge resection:** a nonanatomic operation reserved for patients with limited lung reserve as well as for small peripheral tumors. This definitive therapy is used for poor surgical risk patients or patients with metastatic lesions from sites such as the gastrointestinal tract, head and neck, breast, and genitourinary tract. The physiologic effect following this surgery is minimal, as is the morbidity and mortality. The disadvantage of this operation is a 10–15% recurrence in the lobe left behind (LoCicero, Ponn, and Daly, 2000; LoCicero, 2000).

❖ **Sleeve resection:** performed when tumors are protruding into the main bronchus. If tumors originate in the right upper lobe bronchus where a lobectomy cannot be performed, a resection of the right main and intermediate bronchial sleeve allows for adequate margins around the tumor. Bronchial reanastomosis preserves uninvolved right lower and middle lobes. In the hands of skilled thoracic surgeons, the sleeve resection is becoming more common, thereby limiting the pneumonectomy, which can be compromising.

❖ Video-assisted thoracic surgery (VATS) improves patient care by decreasing the painful recovery period and shortening hospital stays.

   ❖ Procedure:

   1. Surgeon makes 2–4 tiny openings between the ribs while viewing the patient's internal organs on a television monitor (United States Surgical Corporation, 1999). Blebs can be treated, diagnoses and treatments around the lung and heart can be done, and mediastinal tumors can be evaluated.

   2. Ribs are not spread or cut, therefore bone pain is reduced.

   3. Surgical lung sealant, a type of superglue, is used to reduce air leaks at the time of surgery. The sealant is applied with a syringe to the stapled area intraoperatively, and a light source is applied that polymerizes the glue, thus sealing the treated area. Application of the sealant resulted in control of air leaks in 92% of the patients that were treated (Wain et al., 2001).

Postoperative Nursing Care

❖ Postoperative nursing care for the thoracotomy patient should focus on two major areas: pain and pulmonary management.

A. Pain Control

1. Immediately postoperatively, patients are given intravenous (IV) or epidural patient-controlled analgesia (PCA). IV pain medications frequently used are opioid derivative medications (such as morphine) and IV Toradol®. Patients can have spasms as a result of the resection to the intercostal muscles. Toradol®is contraindicated in patients with renal disease and should not be given for greater than 7–10 days. PCA pumps are discontinued when patients are able to take oral medications or until the chest tube is removed.

2. Other adjunct therapies are instituted, such as sitting up in a chair to reduce tension along the suture site and early ambulation to reduce muscle spasms and to promote good pulmonary management.

B. Pulmonary Management

1. Deep breaths and promotion of early ambulation are two early interventions that decrease pulmonary complications (pneumonia and atelectasis). Coughing and deep breaths at least ten times an hour assisted by an incentive spirometer is essential to allowing the functional parenchyma, the alveoli, to expand.

2. Shortness of breath can occur following a pulmonary resection, and over a few months' time, it will slowly resolve. Reassurance to the patient, increased mobility, and adequate pain control will help control for this unpleasant side effect.

Other postoperative care includes:

A. Cardiac Monitoring:

1. All patients having any type of pulmonary resection may be at risk for atrial arrhythmias such as atrial fibrillation (due to the close proximity of the vagus nerve during the intraoperative period). If atrial fibrillation occurs, patients are started on the appropriate beta-blocker to control for rapid ventricular response and to assist the patient back into sinus rhythm. In rare instances, cardioversion may be required.

2. Atrial fibrillation potentates the risk for developing a stroke. For this reason, anticoagulation therapy with Heparin® and then Coumadin® may be indicated if the atrial fibrillation is of new onset or if there is an alternating pattern of atrial fibrillation and sinus rhythm. Typically, a short course of therapy may be indicated at discharge and is usually discontinued at the patient's first postoperative visit.

B. Wound Care

1. Anytime an incision is made, the patient is at risk for a wound infection. Slightly elevated temperature in the first 24 hours postoperative is not unusual. However, high temperatures continuing into postoperative days two or three should be investigated for infection. Patient should have sputum, urine, and blood cultures and the surgical incision inspected for any overt signs of infection. If an organism is identified, then the appropriate antibiotic is prescribed. If the wound requires drainage, then an incision and drainage is performed, and the wound is packed lightly and monitored closely over the patient's hospital course and at the time of discharge. Home-care nursing may need to be arranged to provide additional wound care.

C. Emotional Support

1. Emotional state preoperatively can have great impact on the entire surgical course. Offer patients opportunities to express their thoughts about their disease.

2. Support structures need to be in place prior to the actual surgical day. If necessary, support groups of other patients should be readily available to assist with questions or concerns that may occur during this emotional time.

3. Healthcare personnel should take the time to explain what is involved with the procedure, what to expect postoperatively and at the time of discharge.

Clinical Care Pathways

1. Clinical pathways were developed in an attempt to contain costs in an era of rising healthcare costs and limited resources (Zehr et al., 1998).
2. Pathway implementation has been shown to reduce hospital length of stay and significantly reduce diagnostic testing (Zehr et al., 1998).
3. They benefit patients and their families because clear expectations of what they may expect during the hospital course is offered.

Complications following Surgical Resection

❖ A successful surgical operation can be measured based upon the complication rates.

❖ Major complications usually seen with a lung resection procedure are pulmonary and cardiovascular:
   ❖ Pulmonary complications may include:
      1. Pneumonia
      2. Emphysema
      3. Bronchopulmonary fistulas that may require long-term oxygen therapy, ventilator support, and a long-term hospital stay

- ❖ Cardiovascular complications may include:
    1. Tacharrythmias such as atrial fibrillation that may require medical therapy or cardioversion
    2. Myocardial infarction (MI) is likely to occur if the patient has had an MI within three months of surgery. Cardiac failure, as well as MI, is usually seen in the older patient population group. The 30-day mortality following surgical resection revealed that, as the age of patient increased, the mortality increased. A 70-year-old patient had a mortality rate of 7.1%. The rate is 4.1% for the 60–69-year-old group, and 1.3% for the less than 60-year-old group following a surgical resection (Ginsberg et al., 1983).

Another Therapeutic Modality as an Alternative

Photodynamic Therapy

- ❖ Photodynamic therapy (PDT) shrinks tumors, alleviates symptoms, and offers hope to patients for better quality of life. The future uses of PDT could be for the elderly patient with a cardiac history who is not a surgical candidate or a good nonsurgical option to remove a lung tumor without the surgical and anesthesia risks and high hospital costs.

- ❖ Two-step process: injects a light-activated drug, Photofrin® (porfimer sodium, Sanofi

Pharmaceuticals, Inc., New York, NY) that targets cancer cells. Photofrin selectively concentrates in the cancer cells while largely clearing from healthy tissue (Bruce, 2000). Several days later, the cancerous cells are exposed to a spectrum of light by way of a laser. The light "switches" on the drug, destroying the cancer cells (Bruce, 2000). Photosensitivity begins as soon as the injection occurs and will last for approximately four to six weeks (Bruce, 2000).

❖ Three main contraindications to PDT (Bruce, 2000; Lam, 1994):

1. Known allergies to Photofrin

2. Existing tracheoesophageal or bronchoesophageal fistulas

3. Patients with tumors that are eroding into a major vessel

❖ Other precautionary measures:

1. Caution in patients with endobronchial tumors in which inflammation from the therapy itself can cause obstruction of the patients' airway

2. Esophageal varices are at high risk due to increased incidence of bleeding if PDT is given directly to the varices

3. Caution with other photosensitizing drugs: tetracylcine, phenothiazines, and thiazide diuretics (Bruce, 2000). As there are agents that enhance the effects of Photofrin, there are

agents that decrease the effects, such as Vitamin A compounds, Vitamin E, ethanol, and beta-carotene.

❖ Postoperatively instruct patients to:

1. Protect their skin from photosensitivity and ocular sensitivity (i.e., exposure to UV light) as second and third-degree burns can occur (Bruce, 2000).

2. Wear clothing such as long-sleeved shirts, slacks, gloves, shoes, and socks. Dark sunglasses and a wide brimmed hat are recommended at home. Patients should avoid exposure to strong indoor lighting, close proximity to unshaded light bulbs, and discourage the use of "helmet type" hairdryers. Patients are also told to remain at least six feet from unshielded windows, including automobiles.

8

Chemotherapy

By Judy Phillips, RN, MSN, CCRN, AOCN, FNP-C

Introduction: Advances in Chemotherapy

Chemotherapy regimens have evolved over the years from first generation agents (e.g., mitomycin, ifosfamide, and cisplatin) resulting in 10-15% survival rates at one year, to second generation agents (e.g., cisplatin and etoposide) increasing survival rates to 20-25%. Now third generation regimens, with newer agents usually in combination with a platinum compound, have shown improved treatment outcomes in advanced disease (Frei, 1997; Ramanathan and Belani, 1997; Schiller et al., 2002; NCCN, 2003). They also have shown benefits when combined with other treatment modalities in patients with earlier stage disease (Greco and Hainsworth, 1997; Bunn and Kelly, 1998).

For small cell lung cancer (SCLC), the standard of care has included chemotherapy for both limited and extensive stage disease.

Non-Small Cell Lung Cancer

❖ Platinum-based chemotherapy has been part of standard treatment for advanced NSCLC during the past two decades.

❖ Carboplatin is noted to have a similar mechanism of action with a wide spectrum of activity as cisplatin, but with significantly less toxicity. Less nausea and vomiting, neurotoxicity, ototoxicity, and nephrotoxicity is seen. The need for aggressive hydration is eliminated. However, there is a greater incidence of myelosuppression with carboplatin, most notably thrombocytopenia (Budd et al., 1993; Rapp et al., 1988).

❖ Carboplatin is dosed by looking at renal function along with weight, height, gender, and age. Severe toxicity can occur if renal function is not included. The most commonly used formula is Calvert's formula. Also, glomerular filtration rates are determined by either the Cockcroft and Gault formula (Cockcroft, and Gault, 1976) or Jelliffe's formula (Jelliffe, 1973). See Table 8-1 for these formulas.

New Single Agents for NSCLC

Paclitaxel and Docetaxel
Vinorelbine
Gemcitabine
Irinotecan
Topotecan

❖ All these agents except topotecan demonstrated a 20% or higher response rate with average median survival of about 40 weeks, which was much longer than second-generation cisplatin-based combination regimens.

❖ Trials comparing new chemotherapy agents alone to cisplatin-based combination regimens have occurred. See Tables 8-2, 8-3, and 8-4.

Third Generation Combination Regimen: Paclitaxel-based Combination Regimens have been Studied.

❖ See Tables 8-2 and 8-5

  1. Eastern Cooperative Oncology Group (ECOG) conducted a randomized trial comparing two different doses of paclitaxel with cisplatin to etoposide and cisplatin in previously untreated patients with advanced NSCLC (Bonomi et al., 2000). All patients received cisplatin at $75mg/m^2$ over 24 hours. This was combined with either: Paclitaxel at 250 mg/m^2 with cytokine support or 135 mg/m^2 over 24 hours day 1, or etoposide at 100 mg/m^2 days 1-3. Cycles were repeated every 21 days, and response was evaluated after 2 cycles. 599 patients were enrolled. Results:

    ❖ Response rate was 28%, with one-year survival at 40%, and median survival of 9.9 months with **higher dose paclitaxel and cisplatin.**

- Response rate was 25%, with one-year survival at 37%, and median survival of 9.9 months with **lower dose of paclitaxel and cisplatin.**

- Response rate was 12%, with one-year survival at 7.6%, and median survival of 7.6 months with **etoposide and cisplatin regimen.**

- Quality of life was similar.

2. A second trial looked at Stage IIIB or IV NSCLC with either single-agent cisplatin 100 mg/m^2 or paclitaxel at 175 mg/m^2 over 3 hours with cisplatin 80 mg/m^2. Each regimen was repeated every 21 days. Total of 414 patients were enrolled and randomized. Results:

- Paclitaxel and cisplatin had a 26% response rate. Cisplatin alone had a 17% response rate.

Docetaxel-based Regimens

- Initial combination regimens, evaluated in phase II and III trials, using cisplatin with various docetaxel doses given every 21 days were evaluated. Response rates ranged from 21-48%, with median survival of 8-13 months. The TAX 326 study group (Fossella, 2003) demonstrated comparative overall response, survival, and quality-of-life in combining docetaxel and platinum. See Tables 8-2 and 8-5.

Vinorelbine-based Regimens

- See Tables 8-2, 8-4, and 8-5. These tables outline studies using vinorelbine-based regimens.

Gemcitabine-based Regimens

❖ See Tables 8-2, 8-3, and 8-5. These tables outline studies using gemcitabine-based regimens.

Irinotecan-based Regimens

❖ See Tables 8-2 and 8-5. These tables outline studies using irinotecan-based regimens.

Non-Platinum Combination Regimens

❖ Various non-platinum containing agents continue to be evaluated, including docetaxel and vinorelbine (Miller, 1999), gemcitabine and weekly docetaxel (Spiridonidis et al., 1998), gemcitabine and paclitaxel (Martin et al., 1999), and gemcitabine and vinorelbine (Chen et al., 1999; Barr et al., 1999). Other agents have been used in combination with gemcitabine, including vincristine (Zwitte, Cufer, and Wein, 1999), high dose epirubicin (VanPutten et al., 1999), and topotecan and irinotecan (Cole et al., 1999).

A randomized phase II trial in previously untreated patients with advanced NSCLC compared gemcitabine and docetaxel to docetaxel and cisplatin (Georgoulias et al., 1999). Similar response rates were seen, with 34% responding to gemcitabine and docetaxel and 32% responding to docetaxel and cisplatin. Mean survival times were also similar.

Comparison of Third-Generation Regimens in Advanced Disease

❖ Baseline prognostic variables (stage, weight loss, performance status) predict response to treatment and survival (NCCN, 2003).

❖ Improvements in survival have been noted with newer third-generation regimens, with an average gain of two months for median survival in comparison with historical controls. There are toxicity trade-offs between regimens, with no clear advantage with regards to response rate, survival, or quality-of-life having emerged (Fossella, 2003). See Table 8-5.

❖ For advanced NSCLC second-line therapy (patients who have failed platinum-based regimens), single agent docetaxel is the "standard of comparison" (NCCN, 2003; Fossella et al., 2000; Shepard et al., 2000).

Role of Second-Line Therapy in Advanced Disease

❖ See Table 8-6.

Options for Elderly or Medically Compromised Patients with Advanced Disease

❖ Advanced age is considered an unfavorable prognostic factor in patients with NSCLC. A retrospective analysis of ECOG 5592, however, demonstrated that patients greater than 70 years of age benefited from aggressive platinum-based therapy (Langer et al., 2000). This trial randomized patients to receive cisplatin with etoposide or paclitaxel (low or high dose). Measures of quality of life and efficacy were similar to those of patients less than 70; only leukopenia and neuropsychiatric toxicities were seen more often in the elderly. This trial supports the use of standard third-generation combination regimens for patients with good performance status regardless of age.

❖ Patients who are medically compromised may benefit from monotherapy with gemcitabine, vinorelbine, or a taxane biweekly schedule. Few trials have focused on the medically compromised elderly patient.

Treatment of Unresectable Locally Advanced Disease

❖ Historically, treatment for locally advanced disease has been with radiotherapy; however, several randomized trials have demonstrated the benefit of administering combined chemotherapy sequentially with radiation in patients with unresectable disease (Tables 8-7, 8-8, 8-9).

❖ Toxicities associated with a combination of chemotherapy and radiation modalities, such as pneumonitis and pulmonary fibrosis, can be potentially life-threatening, which should factor into the decision process. To date, there is only one published randomized study comparing concurrent radiation therapy when cytotoxic doses of chemotherapy are used. This European trial evaluated the second-generation regimen of cisplatin, vindesine, and mitomycin (MVP) given concurrently with radiation followed by a 10-day rest period, plus additional radiation versus two courses of MVP followed by continuous thoracic radiation (Furuse et al., 1999). Superior efficacy was seen in the concurrent arm, with a median survival of 16.5 months and a 5-year survival of 16%, compared to a median survival of 13.3 months, and a 5-year survival of 9%. Toxicity profiles were similar with slightly more esophagitis and myelosuppression in the concurrent treatment arm.

Treatment of Early Stage and Resectable Locally Advanced Disease

❖ The role of chemotherapy with or without radiation in early stage NSCLC remains to be defined.

❖ Currently, there is no standard treatment after surgery for locally advanced disease.

❖ During the last two decades, studies evaluating induction or neoadjuvant therapy were conducted using various second-generation chemotherapy regimens plus or minus radiation therapy in patients with potentially resectable locally advanced disease. Response rates have ranged from 40–90% with significant variability in complete resection rates (see Table 8-10). The resection rate variability may be due to lack of surgical staging preoperatively with mediastinoscopy in some trials.

❖ A trial of 69 patients with IIIA or IIIB disease evaluating chemotherapy alone versus chemotherapy and radiation has been published from only one trial to date. The patients received either chemotherapy preoperatively with cisplatin and 5-fluorouracil with radiation (30 Gy), or chemotherapy alone with cisplain, mitomycin, and vinblastine (Fleck et al., 1993). The combined chemotherapy and radiation treatment arm demonstrated a statistically significant advantage over the chemotherapy alone arm with a response rate of 67% versus 44%, and a resectability rate of 52% versus 31%.

Novel Targeted Therapies

❖ Epidermal growth factor receptors (EGFR) have been expressed in many tumors including 40–80% of non-small cell lung cancers, and studies have implicated EGFR with poor prognosis and resistance to chemotherapy (Baselga, 2000; Salomon, et al., 1995).

❖ Monoclonal antibodies, such as C225, are considered anti-EGFR agents or EGFR inhibitors. Monoclonal antibodies attach to the extracellualar ligand binding site, blocking various ligands such as epidermal growth factor or transforming growth factor, which after dimerization activate the intracellualar tyrosine kinase domain.

❖ Tyrosine kinase is the essential first step in signal transduction; it may ultimately lead to increased proliferation, increased metastases, increased angiogenesis, and decreased apoptosis. External approaches with monoclonal antibodies may not eliminate tyrosine kinase activity completely, as various intracellular triggers also exist.

❖ As with administration of other monoclonal antibodies, infusion reactions with C225 may occur.

❖ Other approaches, such as IRESSA, target the intracellular domain and are considered epidermal growth factor receptor-tyrosine kinase inhibitors (EGFR-TKI). These agents completely block activation of tyrosine kinase from both external and internal triggers and activity may be seen in the absence of true overexperession of EGFR.

❖ On May 5, 2003, the FDA approved gefitinib (Iressa) 250 mg tablets as monotherapy treatment for patients with locally advanced or metastatic NSCLC after failure of both platinum-based and docetaxel chemotherapies. Iressa is not recommended for use in combination with chemotherapy. Response rate was found to be 10.6% overall. The 250 mg dosage showed a response rate of 13.6%, whereas a 500 mg dosage was 7.8%; median duration of response was 7%. No benefit was found by adding Iressa to doublet, platinum-based chemotherapy. Iressa should be taken once per day with food. Interstitial lung disease was seen in 1% of patients receiving Iressa, and approximately 1/3 of these 1% were fatal. If acute onset or worsening of pulmonary symptoms occurs, Iressa should be stopped and investigation should occur. Side effects of diarrhea, rash, acne, dry skin, nausea, vomiting, and pruritis have been seen. They have generally been found in the 1st month of treatment and usually were mild (Pazdur, R., 2003).

❖ Trastuzumab, a targeted therapy approved for HER-2/Neu overexpressing breast cancer, may have a role in the treatment of NSCLC as well.

❖ Squamous cell cancers more often express EGFR, while adenocarcinomas are more likely to express HER-2/Neu.

❖ Gene replacement—patients with lung cancer often have p53 deficiency within tumors. P53 is a tumor-suppressor gene that directs repair of damaged DNA or committing a cell to apoptosis. These p53 deficient tumors have demonstrated a lack of responsiveness to chemotherapy and radiation, and it is thought that gene replacement may aid in reversing these and other negative factors. Gene therapy requires a delivery system, and clinical trials have administered p53 either intratumorally or with an adenovirus carrier (Rothe et al., 2000).

❖ RhuMAB VEGF is an anti-vascular endothelial growth factor that serves to inhibit angiogenesis. In NSCLC, patients received paclitaxel and carboplatin alone or with one of two doses of RhuMAB

VEGF (DeVore et al., 2000). There were six massive bleeding episodes, four of which resulted in death.

❖ At ASCO, 2003, Dr. Chavalier presented results of the Randomized International Adjuvant Lung Cancer Trial (IALT) studying cisplatin-based chemotherapy vs. no chemotherapy in 1867 patients with resected NSCLC. IALT was designed to evaluate the impact on survival of 3 to 4 cycles of adjuvant cisplatin-based chemotherapy after complete resection of NSCLC. Overall survival was significantly different and supports adjuvant chemotherapy in resected NSCLC:

	2yr Survival	5 yr Survival	2 yr Disease-Free	5 yr Disease-Free
Chemotherapy:	70%	45%	61%	39%
No Chemotherapy:	67%	40%	55%	34%

Small Cell Lung Cancer

❖ This cancer has a rapid growth rate.

❖ There is a propensity for systemic dissemination and poor treatment outcomes noted with early local or locoregional approaches.

❖ Chemotherapy has been the cornerstone of treatment for both extensive and limited stage disease (refer to Table 8-11).

❖ Standard of care treatment for limited stage disease includes chemotherapy plus thoracic radiation given sequentially, concurrently, or in an alternating manner.

❖ Concurrent treatment offers the advantage of decreasing total treatment time.

❖ Three recent trials employing etoposide and a platinum compound have demonstrated a survival advantage with earlier versus delayed concurrent thoracic radiation therapy (Murray et al., 1993; Goto et al., 1999; Jeremic et al., 1997).

❖ Carboplatin plus etoposide is highly active with response rates ranging between 53–85% in extensive stage disease and between 80–93% in limited stage disease (Ellis et al., 1995; Katakami, et al., 1996; Pfeiffer, Sorenson, and Rose, 1995).

❖ See Table 8-12 for a comparison of carboplatin and cisplatin. The carboplatin plus etoposide arm was associated with significantly less nonhematologic toxicity, and there was a trend toward less hematologic toxicity.

❖ Treatment duration/maintenance therapy: short-term chemotherapy is employed typically with four to six cycles administered. Limiting the number of cycles in less harmful to the marrow, allowing for easier administration of subsequent regimens at the time of progression or relapse.

❖ Dose intensification—Trials evaluating dose intensity have demonstrated increased toxicity with a lack of a survival advantage for increased doses (Crawford et al., 1992; Murray et al., 1999).

❖ Chemotherapy in extensive stage disease: Response rates with cyclophosphamide, doxorubicin, and vincristine triplet or the cisplatin and etoposide doublet has ranged from 51-78%, with median survival times from 8.3 to 9.9 months (Roth et al., 1992; Fukuoka et al., 1991).

❖ Many clinicians currently use carboplatin instead of cisplatin-based combinations for improved tolerability, particularly less nausea, vomiting, and nephrotoxicity (Ellis et al., 1995; Katakami et al., 1996; Kosmidis et al., 1994).

❖ Thoracic radiation has not been found to be helpful in patients with extensive stage disease. See Table 8-13 for activity of newer agents in SCLC.

❖ A study published January 10, 2002 in the New England Journal of Medicine compared irinotecan plus cisplatin with etoposide plus cisplatin for extensive small cell lung cancer. The planned size of the study population was 230 patients, but enrollment was terminated early because an interim analysis found a significant survival improvement of the patients receiving irinotecan plus cisplatin.

❖ Medial survival was 12.8 months in the irinotecan-plus-cisplatin group and 9.4 months in the etoposide-plus-cisplatin group. At two years, the survival with irinotecan-plus cisplatin group was 19.5 percent, whereas the etoposide-plus-cisplatin group was 5.2 percent (Noda et al., 2002).

Treatment of Elderly or Medically Compromised Lung Cancer Patients

❖ Treating these populations is problematic regardless of disease stage. Standard chemotherapy is often poorly tolerated in these patients, particularly with aggressive treatments (i.e., cisplatin).

❖ Frequently, lower doses of chemotherapy or induction chemotherapy are often good.

TABLE 8-1 CARBOPLATIN DOSE CALCULATION

Calvert's formula	Dose (mg) = (target AUCa mg/ml/min)³ (GFR ml/min + 25)
GFR determination	
Cockcroft and Gault formula	Estimated GFR= $\dfrac{\text{ABW in kg } (140 - \text{age})}{\text{Cr} \times 72}$ X 1.0 in males X 0.85 in females
Jelliffe's formula	Estimated GFR: 1) E (males) = ABW 3 (29.305 2[0.203 3 (age]) E (females) = ABW 3 (25.3 2 [0.18 3 (age)]) 2) CrCl = E/(SCr 3 14.4) 3) CrCl/1.73 m2 = CrCl 3 1.73/BSA

aMost 3- to 4-week schedules employ an AUC of 5.0 to 7.5, whereas weekly schedules typically employ an AUC of < = 2.0. AUC = area under time vs. concentration curve; GFR = glomerular filtration rate; ABW = adjusted body weight; SCr = serum creatinine; E = urinary creatinine excretion rate; CrCl = creatinine clearance

TABLE 8-2

Single-Agent Activity of Newer Chemotherapy Agents in NSCLC/Phase I/II Trials

Agent	Number of Studies[a]	Number of Patients	Total CR[b] + PR[b] (%)	Median Survival[c]
Paclitaxel[d,e]	10	317	84 (26%)	37 (24–56)
Docetaxel[f,g]	8	300	77 (26%)	41 (27–48)
Vinorelbine[h]	5	363	126 (35%)	39 (30–52)
Gemcitabine[i,j]	9	572	122 (21%)	41 (31–49)
Irinotecan[k]	4	138	37 (27%)	35 (27–42)
Topotecan[m]	5	119	15 (13%)	38 (33–40)

[a]Number of studies reporting results.

[b]CR = complete response; PR = partial response.

[c]Averaged median survival in weeks (range).

[d]Includes short (1–3 hour) and long (24 hour) infusion durations. No differences in response or survival noted between long and short infusions.

[e]Chang, Kim, Glick, Anderson, Karp, and Johnson, 1993; Murphy, Fossella, Winn, Shin, Hynes, Gross, Davilla, Leimert, Dhingra, Raber, Krakoff, and Kong, 1993; Tan, Herrera, Einzroj, and Wiernik, 1995; Millward, Bishop, Friedlander, Levi, Goldstein, Olver, Smith, Toner, Rischin, and Bell, 1996; Gatzemeier, Heckmeyr, Neuhauss, Schluter, Pawel, Wagner, and Dreps, 1995; Sekine, Nishiwaki, Watanabe, Yoneda, Saijo, and the East Japan Paclitaxel Study Group, 1996; Hainsworth, Thompson, and Greco, 1995; Tester, Jin, Reardon, Cohn, and Cohen, 1997; Akerly, Glantz, Choy, Rege, Sambandam, Joseph, Yee, Rodrigues, Wingate, and Leone, 1998; Ranson, Jayson, Perkins, Anderson, and Thatcher, 1997.

[f]Includes doses ranging between 60 and 100 mg/m². Response rates favored the 75 mg/m² dose level. Survival was similar.

[g]Burris, Eckardt, Fields, Rodriguez, Smith, Thurman, Peacock, Kuhn, Hodges, Bellet, Barssas, LeBail, and Von Hoff, 1993; Cerny, Kaplan, Pavlidis, Schoffski, Epelbaum, van Meerbeeck, Wanders, Franklin, and Kaye, 1994; Fossella, Lee, Murphy, Lippman, Calayag, Pang, Chasen, Shia, Glisson, Benner, Huber, Perez-Soler, Hong, and Raber, 1994; Francis, Rigas, Kris, Pisters, Orazem, Woolley, and Heelan, 1994; Miller, Rigas, Francis, Grant, Pisters, Venkatraman, Woolley, Heelan, and Kris, 1994; Kunitoh, Watanabe, Onoshi, Furuse, Niitani, and Taguchi, 1996; Yokoyama, Kurita, Watanabe, Negoro,

Ogura, Nakano, Minoda, Niitani, and Taguchi, 1994; Kudo, Hino, Fujita, Igarashi, Niitani, and Taguchi, 1994.

[h]Gridelli, Perrone, Gallo, De Marinis, Ianniello, Cigolari, Cariello, Di Costanzo, D'Aprile, Rossi, Migliorino, Bartolucci, Bianco, Pergola, and Monfardini, 1997; Veronesi, Crivellari, Magri, Cartei, Mansutti, Foladore, and Monfardini, 1996; Furuse, Kuba, Yamori, Nakai, Negoro, Katagami, Takada, Kinuwaki, Kawahara, Kubota, Sakuma, and Niitani—for the Japan Vinorelbine Lung Cancer Cooperative Study Group, 1996; Lorusso, Carpagnano, Frasci, Panza, Di Rienzo, Cisternino, Napoli, Orlando, Cinieri, Brunetti, Palazzo, and De Lena, 1995; Furuse, Kubota, Kawahara, Ogawara, Kinuwaki, Montomiya, Nishiwaki, Niitani, and Sakuma, 1994.

[i]Includes various weekly dosing ranges, mostly greater than 800 mg/m2. No clear benefit of dosing > 1000 mg/m^2.

[j]Richards, White, Muss, Powell, Cruz, Andes, Spell, Tarassoff, and Matt, 1994; Fossella, Lippman, Shin, Tarassoff, Calayag-Jung, Perez-Soler, Lee, Murphy, Glisson, Rivera, and Hong, 1997; Abratt, Bezwoda, Falkson, Goedhals, Hacking, and Rugg, 1994; Anderson, Lund, Bach, Thatcher, Walling, and Hansen, 1994; Gatzmeier, Shepherd, LeChevalier, Weynants, Cottier, Groen, Rosso, Mattson, Cortes-Funes, Tonato, Burkes, Gotfried, and Voi, 1996; Nakai, Takada, Yokoyama, Negoro, Kurita, Fukuoka, and Niitani, 1994; LeChevalier, 1996; Perng, Chen, Ming-Liu, Tsai, Lin, Yang, and Whang-Peng, 1997; Manegold, Stahel, Mattson, Ricci, van Valree, Bergman, and ten Bokkel Huinik, 1997.

[k]Fukuoka, Niitani, Suzuki, Motomiya, Hasegawa, Nishiwaki, Kuriyama, Ariyoshi, Negoro, Masuda, Nakajima, and Taguchi, 1992; Negoro, Fukuoka, Niitani, Suzuki, Nakabayashi, Kimura, Motomiya, Kurita, Hasegawa, and Kuriyama, 1991; Baker, Khan, Lynch, Savaraj, Snadler, Feun, Schaser, Hanover, and Petit, 1997; Nakai, Fukuoka, Furuse, Nakao, Yoshimori, Ogura, Hara, Sakata, Saito, and Hascgawa, 1991; Douillard, Ibrahim, Riviere, Spaeth, Chomy, Soussan, and Mathieu-Boue, 1995.

[l]NR = not reported.

[m]Perez-Soler, Glisson, Kane, Lee, Raber, and Hong, 1994; Lynch, Kalish, Strauss, Elias, Skarin, Shulman, Posner, and Freii, 1994; Hochester, Liebes, Speyer, Sorich, Taubes, Oratz, Wernz, Chachoua, Raphael, Vinci, and Blum, 1994; Kindler, Kris, Smith, Slevin, and Krebs, 1997; Perez-Soler, Khuri, Pisters, Robinson, Wimberly, Lee, and Fossella, 1997.

TABLE 8-3

Randomized Trial of Gemcitabine versus Etoposide plus Cisplatin[a]

	Gemcitabine	EC[b]
Number of Patients	26	24
% CR + PR[c]	19%	21%
Median survival (weeks)	37	48
1-year survival	40%	35%
% GR 4 WBC[d]	0	12
% GR 3-4 N, V[e]	4	35

[a]Perng et al., 1997.

[b]E = etoposide, C = cisplatin

[c]CR = complete response, PR = partial response

[d]% GR 4 WBC = % of patients with grade 4 leukopenia

[e]% GR 3-4 N, V = % of patients with grade 3 or 4 nausea and vomiting

TABLE 8-4

Randomized Trial of Single Agent Vinorelbine versus Vinorelbine plus Cisplatin[a]

	Vn[b]	Vn plus C[c]
Number of patients	208	206
% response	14	30
Median survival (weeks)	31	40
% 1-year survival	25	35

[a]LeChevalier et al., 1994.

[b]Vn = vinorelbine

[c]C = cisplatin

TABLE 8-5

Efficacy of Randomized Cooperative Group Trials Comparing Third-Generation Regimens

	SWOG 9509			ECOG 1594		
Regimen	Cb/P	C/Vn	C/P	C/G	C/D	Cb/P
Number of patients	207	201	292	288	289	290
Reponse rate (%)	25	28	21	22	17	15
Median survival (months)	8	8	7.8	8.1	7.4	8.1
1-year survival (%)	38	36	31	36	31	34

C = cisplatin; P = paclitaxel; Cb = carboplatin; Vn = vinorelbine;
G = gemcitabine; D = docetaxel

TABLE 8-6
Single Agents in Second-Line Therapy for Advanced NSCLC

Dose and Schedule	Number of Patients	Overall Response Rate (%)	Median Survival (wks)
P 175 mg/m^2 24 hr q 21 d[a]	40	3	18
P 140 mg/m^2 96 hr q 21 d[b]	11	0	NR
P 135 or 200 mg/m^2 1 hr q 21 d[c]	26	23	NR
D 75 mg/m^2 q 21 d[d]	125	12.2 (P7)	22
V 20 mg/m^2/wk[e]	18	0	NR
CPT-11 200 mg/m^2 q 21–28 d[f]	22	14	NR
G 1000 mg/m^2/wk[g]	30	20	22
MTA 500 mg/m^2 q 21 d[h]	22 (PT)	8	NR
	22 (NP)	35	NR

P = paclitaxel, D = docetaxel, V = vinorelbine, CPT-11 = irinotecan, G = gemcitabine, PT = failed prior platinum containing regimen, NP = failed prior non-platinum containing regimen, MTA = multitargeted antifolate

TABLE 8-6
Single Agents in Second-Line Therapy for Advanced NSCLC (continued)

[a] Murphy et al., 1994.

[b] Socinski and Steagal, 1997.

[c] Hainsworth, Thompson, and Greco, 1995.

[d] Fossella et al., 2000 (TAX 320).

[e] Rinaldi et al., 1994.

[f] Nakai et al., 1991.

[g] Gridelli et al., 1999.

[h] Mattson et al., 1999.

TABLE 8-7
Positive Randomized Trials with Sequential Chemotherapy and
Radiation versus Radiation Alone

Treatment	Number of Patients	MST	2 year Survival	5 year Survival
Radiation[a,b]	77	9.7	13%	6%
OR				
Vn–C–Radiation	78	13.8	26%	17%
Radiation[c,d]	176	10	14%	3%
OR				
Vd–L–CTX–Radiation	176	12	21%	6%
Radiation once daily[a,e]	149	11.4	19%	5%
OR				
Radiation twice daily[f]	152	12.3	24%	6%
OR				
V–C–Radiation[a]	151	13.8	32%	8%

MST = Mean survival time in months, V = vinblastine, C = cisplatin,
Vn = vindesine, L = lomustine, CTX = cyclophosphamide.

[a]60 Gy over 6 weeks.

[b]Dillman et al., 1990.

[c]65 Gy over 45 days.

[d]LeChevalier et al., 1991.

[e]Sause et al., 1995.

[f]69 Gy given as 1.2 Gy twice daily 5 days per week.

TABLE 8-8
Phase I/II Single-Agent Trials as Radiosensitization

Dose Schedule/ Maximum Tolerance Dose	Radiation Therapy Schedule	Toxicity
P 60 mg/m^2 weekly × 6 weeks[a]	60 Gy in 2 Gy FX over 6 weeks	esophagitis/ pneumonitis
D 30 mg/m^2 weekly × 6 weeks[b]	64 Gy in 2 Gy FX over 6.5 weeks	esophagitis
G 1000 mg/m^2 weekly × 6 weeks[c,d]	60 Gy in 2 Gy FX over 6 weeks	pulmonary toxicity severe esophagitis
CPT-11 60 mg/m^2 weekly × 6 weeks[e]	60 Gy in 2 Gy FX over 6 weeks	esophagitis pneumonitis diarrhea

P = paclitaxel, D = docetaxel, G = gemcitabine, CPT-11 = irinotecan, FX = fraction

[a]Choy et. al. 1994; Choy et al., 1998.

[b]Koukourakis et al., 1999.

[c]Scalliet et al., 1998.

[d]Study closed early due to treatment related deaths/excessive toxicity.

[e]Kudoh et al., 1996.

TABLE 8-9
Phase I/II Doublet Trials as Radiosensitization

Recommended Dose/Schedule	Radiation Schedule	Toxicity
P 50 mg, 1 hr + Cb AUC 2 Weekly × 7 then Consolidation with P 200 mg/m^2 + Cb AUC 6 q 21 Days × 2[a]	66 Gy in 2 Gy FX over 7 weeks	esophagitis pneumonitis
P 35 mg/m^2, 1 hr Twice weekly and Cb AUC 1.5 Weekly × 6 then Consolidation with P 200 mg/m^2 + Cb AUC 6 q 21 Days × 2[b]	FX twice daily	esophagitis neutropenia
C 80 mg/m^2 day 1 + Vn 15 mg/m^2 days 1,8 Both every 21 days × 2[c]	60 Gy in 2 Gy FX over 6 weeks	esophagitis myelosuppression

P = paclitaxel, Cb = carboplatin, C = cisplatin, Vn = vinorelbine,
FX = fraction
[a]Choy et al., 1998.
[b]Lau et al., 1999.
[c]Masters et al., 1998.

TABLE 8-10
Selected Phase II Trials of Chemotherapy or Chemoradiation in Potentially Resectable Stage III Disease

Treatment	Number of Patients	Response Rate	Complete Resection	Median Survival	Long-Term Survival
CTX-A-P[a]	41	43	88	32 months	31%, 3-year
Vd-E-C[b]	21	70	14	8 months	34%, 1-year
M-V-C[c]	136	78	65	19 months	17%, 5-year
C-F-L[d]	34	65	62	18 months	18%, 4-year
V-C[e]	74	64	31	15 months	23%, 3-year
C-F/C-E-F	85	92 (Includes SD)	71	NR	40%, 3-year
Split RT (40 Gy)[f]					
I-Cb-E × 2, Then E-C/	54	69	63	NR	30%, 3-year
HfRT (45 Gy)[g]					

TABLE 8-10
Selected Phase II Trials of Chemotherapy or Chemoradiation in Potentially Resectable Stage III Disease (continued)

Treatment	Number of Patients	Response Rate	Complete Resection	Median Survival	Long-Term Survival
45 Gy)[g]					
C-V-F × 2/	42	74	81	NR	37%, 5-year
HfRT					
(42 Gy)[h]					

CTX = cytoxan, A = doxorubicin, C = cisplatin, Vd = vindesine, E = etoposide, M = mitomycin, V = velban, F = 5-fluorouracil, L = leucovorin, I = ifosfamide, Cb = carboplatin, RT = radiation therapy, hfRT = hyperfractionated radiation therapy, SD = stable disease, NR = not reported.

[a]Skarin et al., 1989.
[b]Bitran et al., 1986.
[c]Martini et al., 1993.
[d]Elias et al., 1997.
[e]Sugarbaker et al., 1995.
[f]Faber et al., 1989.
[g]Thomas et al., 1999.
[h]Choi et al., 1997.

TABLE 8-11
Commonly Used Combination Chemotherapy Regimens for the
Treatment of Small Cell Lung Cancer

(Postmus, and Smit, 1998)

Regimen	Dose (mg/m²)	Schedule
CDE		
Cyclophosphamide	1,000	Day 1
Doxorubicin	45	Day 1
Etoposide	100	Days 1–5
EP[a]		
Cisplatin	80	Day 1
Etoposide	120	Days 1–3
CAV		
Cyclophosphamide	1,000	Day 1
Adriamycin	50	Day 1
Vincristine	1.4	Day 1
(V)ICE		
(Vincristine)	(1.4)	Day 14
Ifosfamide	5,000	Day 1
Carboplatin	300	Day 1
Etoposide	180	Days 1 & 2

[a]Especially suitable for combination with concurrent thoracic radiotherapy.

TABLE 8-12
Phase III Randomized Trial Results Comparing Etoposide Plus
Carboplatin to Etoposide Plus Cisplatin

Regimen[a]	Number of Patients	Overall Response	Complete Response	Median survival
		N (%)	N (%)	months
Cb—300 mg/m² IV d 1	LD: 41	35 (86)	15 (37)	11.8
E—100 mg/m²/d IV d 1–3	ED: 31	20 (64)	5 (16)	11.8
Cycle = 21 days				
C—50 mg/m²/d IV d 1–2	LD: 41	30 (73)	18 (44)	12.5
E—100 mg/m²/d IV d 1–3	ED: 30	15 (50)	3 (10)	12.5
Cycle = 21 days				

Trial completed by the Hellenic Oncology Group.

Cb = carboplatin, E = etoposide, C = cisplatin, IV = intravenously,
LD = limited-stage disease, ED = extensive-stage disease.

[a]Patients with LD at the end of the third cycle were eligible to receive
concurrent thoracic radiation with the fourth cycle of chemotherapy (Dose
35 Gy). Patients with LD who achieved a complete response received
prophylactic cranial irradiation (Dose 20 Gy).

TABLE 8-13
Activity of Newer Agents in SCLC

Agent	Untreated Patients	Sensitive Disease[a]	Resistant Disease[b]
Paclitaxel	+	+	+
Docetaxel	+	+	?
Gemcitabine	+	?	+
Topotecan	+	+	2
Irinotecan	+	+	2
Vinorelbine	+	?	?

Table reproduced from Postmus and Smit, 1998.

[a]Sensitive disease is from tumor progression after response of greater than 3 months duration.

[b]Resistant disease is tumor progression during first-line therapy or after response of less than 3 months duration.

9

Radiation Therapy

Introduction

❖ Radiotherapy is an integral component of treatment for lung cancer, especially with combined modality. The goal is to irradiate the target structures, yet minimize incidental irradiation of non-target structures like the heart, spinal cord, or brachial plexus.

❖ Successful outcomes of radiotherapy depends on:
  ❖ A clear definition of target volume
  ❖ The optimal radiation dose and fractionation schedules
  ❖ A proper radiation portal arrangement to secure the optimal dose distribution within the target volume (Choi, 2000)

❖ In an attempt to enhance local disease control and have less normal tissue toxicity, new innovative treatment approaches being investigated are:

- ✦ Radiation dose escalation
- ✦ Altered fractionation schedules
- ✦ Improvements in radiation dose distribution
- ✦ Brachytherapy procedures using radioactive seeds
- ✦ Use of radioprotectors (i.e., amifostine) and chemoradiation schemes

- ❖ Other measures to overcome hypoxic tumor cells under investigation are:

  - ✦ High linear energy transfer (LET) beams
  - ✦ Radiotherapy under hyperbaric conditions
  - ✦ The use of hypoxic cell sensitizers
  - ✦ Hyperthermia (Choi, 2000)

Standard Therapy—Non-Small Cell Lung Cancer

- ❖ Radiotherapy (RT) is an important component of treatment of non-small cell lung cancer (NSCLC). RT is used extensively in the definitive and post-operative setting, and more recently in trials evaluating preoperative treatment. Individuals with NSCLC who are appropriate candidates for RT fall into one of the following categories:

  a. Medically inoperable Stage I and II NSCLC— commonly seen in patients with extensive tobacco histories. Most have other smoking-related diseases, such as coronary artery disease, chronic obstructive pulmonary disease, and peripheral vascular disease, which render them inoperable even though definitive resection might be indicated.

b. Unresectable Stage III NSCLC—advanced local disease in the thoracic cavity.

c. Postoperative therapy in Stages II and III NSCLC—for positive or close surgical margins or lymph node involvement.

d. Superior pulmonary sulcus tumor—presenting in the apex of the lung, and is usually unresectable secondary to its proximity to a number of critical structures.

e. Metastatic spread of disease—outside the thoracic cavity (i.e., brain, bone, adrenal gland); usually treated with palliative therapy.

f. Recurrent disease—includes endobronchial lesions that obstruct the bronchi.

Primary Radiation Therapy

❖ Medically inoperable patients with early stage disease (Stage I and II) are usually offered RT with or without chemotherapy.

❖ RT covers the primary lesion and regional lymphatics to a dose of 50–65 Gy over a five-to-six-week period.

❖ Stage IIIA or IIIB NSCLC can receive RT to doses of 50–65 Gy using daily fractionation over a five-to-six-week period of time. Randomized trials have compared standard daily radiotherapy (60 Gy) with twice-daily treatment of a higher dose (69.6 Gy) and with an accelerated regimen that delivered 54 Gy over 2.5 weeks. Both altered fractionation schedules resulted in improved survival (Khuri, Keller, and Wagner, 1999).

❖ Introducing combined chemotherapy and radiotherapy has improved outcomes in Stage III disease. Current approaches include induction chemotherapy for several cycles followed by radiotherapy or concurrent chemoradiation. Cisplatin, vinblastine, carboplatin, and paclitaxel have all been used in these trials. Radiotherapy is usually given in a dose of 50 to 60 Gy over 5–6 weeks.

❖ *In advanced disease (Stage IV), patient care is individualized and usually palliative. The goal of treatment is to relieve symptoms, including shortness of breath, airway obstruction, pain, or neurologic symptoms. The primary site is treated with radiotherapy consisting of 30 Gy over a two-week period. Bone, brain, and adrenal metastasis may also be treated with short courses of palliative radiotherapy (8–30 Gy).

Preoperative Radiation Therapy

❖ Preoperative RT with or without chemotherapy has been used for patients with Stage III disease.

❖ Advantages: tumors are better-oxygenated and better-vascularized. Research from the Cleveland Clinic shows promising results in terms of tumor response, disease control, survival, and toxicity after short-course induction chemoradiotherapy and surgical resection in patients with Stage III disease. Patients received 12-day induction therapy of a 96-hour continuous infusion of cisplatin (20 mg/m2 per day), 24-hour infusion of paclitaxel (175 mg/m2), and concurrent accelerated fractionation radiotherapy (1.5 Gy twice daily) to a dose of 30 Gy, followed by surgical resection 4 weeks later and a second postoperative identical course of chemotherapy and concurrent radiotherapy (30–33 Gy). This regimen resulted in good tumor response and downstaging, with 71% of those who underwent thoracotomy able to be resected for cure. Thirty-one patients were downstaged to mediastinal node negative (Stage 0, I, or II) status. The median survival was modestly improved compared with historical controls. Induction toxicity resulted in hospitalization of 18 (40%) patients for neutropenic fever (Rice et al., 1998).

Postoperative Radiation Therapy

❖ Stage I and II disease receive postoperative adjuvant therapy in patients with close or positive margins, or N1 or N2 disease. However, the appropriate role of postoperative radiotherapy remains ill-defined despite a number of randomized trials.

Endobronchial Brachytherapy

❖ Endobronchial occlusion is a common and potentially life-threatening complication.

❖ Endobronchial RT is used to palliate symptoms arising from partial airway obstruction (Khuri, Keller, and Wagner, 1999). In palliative care, 50–100% of patients have reported symptomatic relief. Studies also report that two-thirds to three-quarters of the remainder of the patient's life is symptom improved or symptom free (Mehta, 1996).

Standard Treatment—Small Cell Lung Cancer

❖ RT is primarily used in small cell lung cancer (SCLC) in a palliative setting for sites of metastatic disease including skeletal and brain metastasis.

❖ There are a number of clinical trials evaluating the role of radiotherapy in aggressive chemoradiation protocols and in the prevention of brain metastasis (prophylactic cranial irradiation [PCI]).

New Technologies

❖ Major advances in technology have significantly impacted the planning and delivery of RT and have resulted in increased selectivity of irradiation to the tumor and a decrease in the dose to the normal tissues and critical structures:

1. 3-D Treatment Planning: Unlike conventional planning, utilizing three dimensional conformal treatment planning allows higher doses to be administered, while sparing the surrounding structures (Marks and Sibley, 1999; Graham, 2001). Historically, radiation fields were directly anteriorly, posteriorly, laterally, or simple obliques. Now with the computer-assisted transfer of complex three-dimensional geometric information, field shaping and blocking has become more highly defined, and more unusual beams can be directed towards just the target structure (Tubiana and Eschwedge, 2000).

   a. In the past, 60-66 Gy, over $6^1/_2$ weeks, delivering 2 Gy a day was the standard with conventional planning, but now 70–73 Gy with 3-D planning can be obtained. However, escalation of dose is still under investigation. Without 3-D planning, radiation oncologists often make the field larger than it might need to be in order to compensate for uncertainties in the definition of the target volume, thus potentially increasing acute and long term toxicities.

2. Intensity Modulated Radiation (IMRT): Relatively new and fancy method to deliver radiation. In order to understand this, it's best

to first review conventional radiation techniques. With conventional approaches, the entire target volume is typically included within each of the radiation fields. While the dose to each region of the tumor from each field is not necessarily constant, each region of the target generally does receive a significant dose from each conventionally-designed treatment beam. With IMRT, this is no longer true. Each radiation beam has its own intensity map. Using a multi-leaf collimator, IMRT produces a highly complex, tightly conforming dose and dose-rate gradient that is distributed around target volumes and modulated to the irregularities of the target volume. With IMRT, more complex conformal fields are targeted to the tumor, allowing a potentially more homogeneous and differentiated dose distribution delivered to the tumor (Tubiana and Eschwège, 2000).

3. **Multimodality Radiation and Chemotherapy:** Concurrent chemotherapy and radiotherapy may be one of the most beneficial strategies to improve response and prolong survival in patients with either advanced resectable or unresectable disease (Mach et.al., 1999). Rationales for combining chemotherapy and radiotherapy include:

   a. The independent action of each modality, which enhances the overall effectiveness and improves survival rates.

    b. Toxicity independence, which allows delivery of the full dose of each modality without additive toxicity.

    c. Cytoprotection of normal tissues possible with radioprotective and chemoprotective agents, which allows higher doses of radiotherapy to be delivered. Agents such as Amifostine used in conjunction with radiation therapy (2Gy/day, total dose 60gy, with 340 mg/m 2 15 minutes prior to RT) prevents pneumonitis or esophagitis later. (Antonadou, 1999).

    d. Chemosensitization or enhancement, which certainly helps local control.

4. Particle Beam Radiation Therapy: Proton beam therapy uses protons to fight cancer. Protons are stable, positively charged subatomic particles with a mass 1800 times that of an electron. These characteristics allow the proton's dose of radiation to be released at an exact shape and depth within the body (Optivus Technology, 2000). Proton beam radiation is unlike megavoltage X-rays in that it has weight and mass, and usually an electrical charge. This type of radiation includes parts of atoms such as negative electron or beta particles, positively charged protons, and neutral neutrons. Massive cyclotrons and linear accelerators that use enormous amounts of energy are used to accelerate these particles. Proton beams have been used for treatment since the mid-1950s, but for most of that time, they were used only in physics laboratories. Proton therapy provides the radiation oncologist with a highly precise method of placing radiation within a patient when compared with conventional radiotherapy using megavoltage X-rays (photons) or electrons (Bush et. al, 1999b).

10

Key Clinical Implications of Standard Treatment Modalities

Key Clinical Points

❖ Lung cancer should be suspected in patients who have symptoms caused by either local or systemic effects of the tumor or who have an abnormal chest radiograph.

❖ Patients with lung cancer should be assessed by a multidisciplinary team, including a thoracic surgeon, medical oncologist, radiation oncologist, and possibly a pulmonoligist.

❖ Patients with enlarged lymphopathy (>1cm) in the mediastinum visible on CT should have further evaluation prior to surgical resection (Silvestri, Tanoue, Margolis, Barker, and Detterbeck, 2003).

❖ Patients who seek thoracic surgery should not be necessarily concerned with age, but more with their functional status and co-morbidities related to cardiac and pulmonary dysfunctions.

❖ If patients are being considered for lung cancer
resection, spirometry should be performed.
Patients are at risk if their FEV1 is less than 0.7 L
and/or 40% predicted. (Reilly, 1999). A patient's
DLCO should be greater than 60% predicted.

❖ NCSLC: Stage I and II cancers are, by definition,
localized to the lung itself and the mainstay of
treatment has traditionally been surgical resection. Stage IIIA and B tumors are localized to the
chest, involving the lung and mediastinal lymph
nodes. The mediastinal nodes cannot be easily
resected with a margin of normal tissue, therefore
the traditional approach has primarily been radiotherapy. Unfortuntately, there is no clear consen-
sus of which optimal neoadjuvant and adjuvant
chemotherapy regimens should be utilized.
Ongoing trials include paclitaxel, docetaxel, gemcitabine, and vinorelbine. Other agents being
studied in combination protocols are 5-fluo-
rouracil, carboplatin, cisplatin, cyclophosphamide,
doxorubicin, etoposide, ifosfamide, mitomycin C,
teniposide, uracil + tegafur, vinblastine, vincristine, and vindesine.

❖ SCLC: differing in the site of their genetic damage, the growth is quick and spreads to the lymph
nodes and other organs earlier than NCSLC. SCLC
initially is more responsive to chemotherapy.
Chemotherapy is typically given in four to six
cycles, usually in combination. Established agents
are carboplatin, cisplatin, cyclophosphamide,

doxorubicin, etoposide, ifosfamide, methotrexate, teniposide, and vincristine. New agents include docetaxel, gemcitabine, irinotecan, paclitaxel, topotecan, and vinorelbine.

❖ A platinum based doublet chemotherapy remains standard treatment for metastic lung cancer

❖ Targeted therapy such as Iressa appears promising in the treatment of lung cancer

❖ New evidence suggests that chemotherapy may be effective as adjuvant treatment to surgery for early stage lung cancer.

❖ Radiation therapy uses X-rays or other high-energy rays to kill cancer cells and shrink tumors. Radiation therapy can be used alone or in addition to surgery and/or chemotherapy.

❖ Radiation therapy may also be used to prevent the cancer from growing in the brain, commonly referred to as prophylactic cranial irradiation (PCI).

References: Chapters 6–10

Abratt, R., Bezwoda, W., Falkson, G., Goedhals, L., Hacking, D., and Rugg, T. (1994). Efficacy and safety profile of gemcitabine in non-small cell lung cancer: A Phase II study. *Journal of Clinical Oncology,* 12(8):1535–1540.

Abratt, R., Hacking, D., Goedhals, L., and Bezwoda, W. (1997). Weekly gemcitabine and monthly cisplatin for advanced non-small cell lung cancer. *Seminars in Oncology,* 24(3, Suppl. 8): 8–23.

Abratt, R., Sandler, A., Crino, L., Steward, W., Shepherd, F., Green, M., Nguyen, B., and Peters, G. (1998). Combined cisplatin and gemcitabine for non-small cell lung cancer: Influence of scheduling on toxicity and drug delivery. *Seminars in Oncology,* 25(4, Suppl. 9):35–43.

Akerly, W., Glantz, M., Choy, H., Rege, V., Sambandam, S., Joseph, P., Yee, L., Rodrigues, B., Wingate, P., and Leone, L. (1998). Phase II trial of weekly paclitaxel in advanced non-small cell lung cancer. *Journal of Clinical Oncology,* 16(1):153–158.

Alexander, J. and Anderson, R. (2000). Preoperative cardiac evaluation of the thoracic surgical patient and management of perioperative cardiac events. In: Shields, T. W., LoCicero, J., and Ponn, R. *General Thoracic Surgery,* 5th ed. (pp. 305–313). Philadelphia: Lippincott Williams and Wilkins.

Anderson, H., Lund, B., Bach, F., Thatcher, N., Walling, J., and Hansen, H. (1994). Single agent activity of weekly gemcitabine in advanced non-small cell lung cancer: A Phase II study. *Journal of Clinical Oncology,* 12(9):1821–1826.

Baker, L., Khan, R., Lynch, T., Savaraj, N., Sandler, A., Feun, L., Schaser, R., Hanover, C., and Petit, R. (1997). Phase II study of irinotecan (CPT-11) in advanced non-small cell lung cancer (NSCLC). *Proceedings of the American Society of Clinical Oncology,* 16:1658.

Barr, F., Mirsky, H., Clinthorne, D., Bendel, S., and Smith, F. (1999). Phase III study of gemcitabine and vinorelbine salvage chemotherapy for taxane-resistant non-small cell lung cancer (NSCLC). *Proceedings of the American Society of Clinical Oncology,* 18:1914.

Basalga, J. (2000). New technologies in epidermal growth factor receptor-targeted cancer therapy. An overview of novel theapeutic agents in development. *Signal,* 1:12–21.

Beckles, M., Sprio, S., Colice, G., and Rudd, R. (2003a). The physiologic evaluation of patients with lung cancer being considered for resectional surgery. *Chest,* 123(1): 105-113.

Beckles, M., Sprio, S., Colice, G., and Rudd, R. (2003b). Initial evluation of the patient with lung cancer. *Chest,* 123(1): 97-104.

Belani, C. (1999). Docetaxel (Taxotere) in combination with platinum-based regimens in non-small cell lung cancer: Results and future developments. *Seminars in Oncology,* 26(3, Suppl. 10):15–18.

Bitran, J., Golomb, H., Hoffman, P., Albain, K., Evans, R., Little, A., Purl, S., and Skosey, C. (1986). Protochemotherapy in non-small cell lung carcinoma. An attempt to increase surgical respectability and sur-vival. A preliminary report. *Cancer,* 57(1):44–53.

Bonomi, P., Kim, K., Fairclough, D., Cella, D., Kugler, J., Rowinsky, E., Jiroutek, M., and Johnson, D. (2000). Comparison of survival and quality of life in advanced non-small cell lung cancer patients treated with two dose levels of paclitaxel combined with cisplatin ver-sus etoposide with cisplatin: Results of an Eastern Cooperative Oncology Group trial. *Journal of Clinical Oncology,* 18(3):623–631.

Bruce, S. (2000). Photodynamic therapy: Another option in cancer treatment. *Clinical Journal of Oncology Nursing,* 5(3): 95–99.

Bush, D.A., Dunbar, R.D., Bonnet, R., Slater, J.D., Cheek, G.A., and Slater, J.M. (1999a). Pulmonary injury from proton and conventional radiotherapy as revealed by CT. *AJR-American Journal of Roentgenology,* 172(3): 735–739.

Budd, G., Ganapathi, R., Bauer, L., Murthy, S., Adelstein, D., Gibson, V., McLain, D., Sergi, J., and Burkewski, R.

(1993). Phase I study of WR-2721 and carboplatin. *European Journal of Cancer*, 29A(8):1122–1127.

Bunn, P. and Kelly, K. (1998). New chemotherapeutic agents prolong survival and improve quality of life in non-small cell lung cancer: A review of the literature and future directions. *Clinical Cancer Research*, 4(5):1087–1100.

Burris, H., Eckardt, J., Fields, S., Rodriguez, G., Smith, L., Thurman, A., Peacock, N., Kuhn, J., Hodges, S., Bellet, R., Bayssas, M., LeBail, N., and Von Hoff, D. (1993). Phase II trials of Taxotere in patients with non-small cell lung cancer. *Proceedings of the American Society of Clinical Oncology*, 12:335.

Bush, D.A., Slater, J.D., Bonnet, R., Cheek, G.A., Dunbar, R.D., Moyers, M., and Slater, J.M. (1999b). Proton-beam radiotherapy for early-stage lung cancer. *Chest*, 116(5): 1313–1319.

Cerny, T., Kaplan, S., Pavlidis, N., Schoffski, P., Epelbaum, R., van Meerbeeck, J., Wanders, J., Franklin, H., and Kaye, S. (1994). Docetaxel (Taxotere) is active in non-small cell lung cancer: A phase II trial of the EORTC early clinical trials group (LCTG). *British Journal of Cancer*, 70(2):384–387.

Chang, A., Kim, K., Glick, J., Anderson, T., Karp, D., and Johnson, D. (1993). Phase II study of Taxol, merbarone and piroxantrone in stage IV non-small cell lung cancer: The Eastern Cooperative Oncology Groups results. *Journal of the National Cancer Institute*, 85(5):388–394.

Chen, Y., Whang-Peng, J., Perng, R., Liu, T., Yang, K., Lin, W., Wu, H., Shih, J., Liu, J., Chen, L., and Tsai, C. (1999). A multicenter phase II study of gemcitabine and vinorelbine in patients with advanced stage IIIB/IV NSCLC. *Proceedings of the American Society of Clinical Oncology*, 17:1856.

Choi, N.C. (2000). Cancer of the intrathorax. In: C.C. Wang (ed.). *Clinical Radiation Oncology: Indications, Techniques, and Results,* 2nd ed. (pp. 295–333). New York: Wiley-Liss.

Choi, N., Carey, R., Daly, W., Mathisen, D., Wain, J., Wright, C., Lynch, T., Grossbard, M., and Grillo, H. (1997). Potential impact on survival of improved tumor downstaging and resection rate by preoperative twice-daily radiation and concurrent chemotherapy in stage IIIA non-small cell lung cancer. *Journal of Clinical Oncology,* 15(2):712–722.

Choy, H., Akerley, W., Safran, H., Clark, J., Rege, V., Papa, A., Glantz, M., Putawala, Y., Soderberg, C., and Leone, L. (1994). Phase I trial of outpatient weekly paclitaxel and concurrent radiation therapy for advanced non-small cell lung cancer. *Journal of Clinical Oncology,* 12(12):2682–2686.

Choy, H., Safran, H., Akerley, W., Graziano, S., Bogart, J, and Cole, B. (1998). Phase II trial of weekly paclitaxel and concurrent radiation therapy for locally advanced non-small cell lung cancer. *Clinical Cancer Research,* 4(8):1931–1936.

Choy, H., Shyr, Y., Cmelak, A., Mohr, P., and Johnson, D. (2000). Patterns of practice survey for non-small cell lung cancer in the U. S. *Cancer,* 88(6):1336–1346.

Cockcroft, D. and Gault, M. (1976). Prediction of creatinine clearance from serum creatinine. *Nephron,* 16(1):31–41.

Cole, J., Rinaldi, D., Lormand, N., Brierre, J., Barnes, B., Fontenot, M., Buller, E., and Rainey, J. (1999). A phase I-II trial of topotecan and gemcitabine for patients with previously treated advanced non-small cell lung cancer (NSCLC). *Proceedings of the American Society of Clinical Oncology,* 18:1927.

Crawford, J., Ozer, H., Stoller, R., Johnson, D., Lyman, G., Tabbara, I., Kris, M., Grous, J., Picozzi, V., Rausch, G., Smith, R., Gradishar, W., Yahanda, A., Vincent, M., Stewart, M., and Glaspy, J. (1991). Reduction by granulocyte colony-stimulating factor of fever and neutropenia induced by chemotherapy in patients with small cell lung cancer. *New England Journal of Medicine,* 325(3):164–170.

DeVore, R., Fehrenbacher, L., Herbst, R., Langer, C., Kelly, K., Gaudreault, J., Holmgren, E., Novotny, W., and Kabbinavar, F. (2000). A randomized phase II trial comparing rhumab VEGF (recombinant humanized monoclonal antibody to vascular endothelial growth factor) plus carboplatin/paclitaxel (CP) to CP alone in patients with stage IIIB/IV NSCLC. *Proceedings of the American Society of Clinical Oncology,* (19):1896.

Dillman, R., Seagren, S., Propert, K., Guerra, J., Eaton, W., Perry, M., Carey, R., Frei, E. 3rd, and Green, M. (1990). A randomized trial of induction chemotherapy plus high-dose radiation versus radiation alone in stage III non-small cell lung cancer. *New England Journal of Medicine,* 323(15):940–945.

Douillard, J., Ibrahim, N., Riviere, A., Spaeth, D., Chomy, P., Soussan, K., and Mathieu-Boue, A. (1995). Phase II study of CPT-11 in patients with non-small cell lung cancer. *Proceedings of the American Society of Clinical Oncology,* 13:363.

Elias, A., Skarin, A., Leong, T., Mentzer, S., Strauss, G., Lynch, T., Shulman, L., Jacobs, C., Abner, A., Baldini, E., Frei, E. 3rd, and Sugarbaker, D. (1997). Neoadjuvant therapy for surgically staged IIIA N2 non-small cell lung cancer. *Lung Cancer,* 17(1):147–161.

Ellis, P., Talbot, D., Priest, K., Jones, A., and Smith I. (1995). Dose intensification of carboplatin and etoposide as first-line combination chemotherapy in small cell lung cancer. *European Journal of Cancer,* 31A(11):1888–1889.

Faber, L., Kittle, C., Warren, W., Bonomi, P., Taylor, S. 4th, Reddy, S., and Lee, M. (1989). Preoperative chemotherapy and irradiation for stage III non-small cell lung cancer. *Annals of Thoracic Surgery,* 47(5):669–677.

Fleck, J., Camargo, J., Godoy, D., Teixeira, P., Braga Filho, A., Barietta, A, and Ferreira, P. (1993). Chemoradiation therapy (CRT) vs. chemotherapy (CT) alone as neoadjuvant treatment for stage III non-small cell lung cancer (NSCLC): Preliminary report of a phase III prospective randomized trial. *Proceedings of the American Society of Clinical Oncology,* 12:333.

Fossella, F., DeVore, R., Kerr, R., Crawford, J., Natale, R., Dunphy, F., Kalman, L., Miller, V., Lee, J. S., Moore, M., Gandara, D., Karp, D., Vokes, E., Kris, M., Kim, Y., Gamza, F., Hammershaimb, L., and the TAX 320 NSCLC Study Group. (2000). Randomized phase III trial of docetaxel versus vinorelbine or ifosfamide in patients with advanced non-small-cell lung cancer previously treated with platinum-containing chemotherapy regimens. *Journal of Clinical Oncology,* 18(12):235–236.

Fossella, F., DeVore, R., Kerr, R., Crawford, J., Natale, R., Dunphy, F., Kalman, L., Gandara, D., Gamza, F., Hammershaimb, L., Kim, Y., and Crist, W. (1999). Phase III trial of docetaxel 100 mg/sqm or 75 mg/sqm versus vinorelbine/ifosfamide for NSCLC previously treated with platinum-based chemotherapy. *Proceedings of the American Society of Clinical Oncology,* 18:1776.

Fosella, F., Lee, J., Murphy, W., Lippman, S., Calayag, M., Pang, A., Chasen, M., Shin, D., Glisson, B., Benner, S., Huber, M., Perez-Soler, R., Hong, W., and Raber, M.

(1994). Phase II study of docetaxel for recurrent or metastatic non-small cell lung cancer. *Journal of Clinical Oncology,* 12(6):1238–1244.

Fosella, F., Lippman, S., Shin, D., Tarassoff, P., Calayag-Jung, M., Perez-Soler, R., Lee, J., Murphy, W., Glisson, B., Rivera, E., and Hong, W. (1997). Maximum tolerated dose defined for single agent gemcitabine: A phase I dose escalation study in advanced chemotherapy naïve patients with non-small cell lung cancer. *Journal of Clinical Oncology,* 15(1):310–316.

Fossella, F., Pereira, J., von Pawel, J., Pluzanska, A., Gorbounova, V., Kaukel, E., Mattson, K., Ramlau, R., Szczęsna, A., Fidias, P., Millward, M., and Belani, C. (2003). Randomized, multinational, phase III study of docetaxel plus platinum combinations versus vinorelbine plus cisplatin for advanced non-small-cell lung cancer: The TAX 326 study group. *Journal of Clinical Oncology,* 21(16):1–9.

Francis, P., Rigas, J., Kris, M., Pisters, K., Orazem, J., Woolley, K., and Heelan, R. (1994). Phase II trial of docetaxel in patients with stage III and IV non-small cell lung cancer. *Journal of Clinical Oncology,* 12(6):1232–1237.

Frei, E. III. (1997). Non-small cell lung cancer: Novel treatment strategies. *Chest,* 112(4, Suppl.): 266S–268S.

Fry, W. (2000). Thoracic incisions. In: Shields, T. W., LoCicero, J., and Ponn, R. *General Thoracic Surgery,* 5th ed. (pp. 367–374). Philadelphia: Lippincott Williams and Wilkins.

Fukuoka, M. and Masuda, N. (1994). Clinical studies of irinotecan alone and in combination with cisplatin. *Cancer Chemotherapy and Pharmacology,* 34: S105–S111.

Fukuoka, M., Furuse, K., Saijo, N., Nishiwaki, Y., Ikegami, H., Tamura, T., Shimoyama, M., and Suemasu, K. (1991).

Randomized trial of cyclophosphamide, doxorubicin, and vincristine versus cisplatin and etoposide versus alternation of these regimens in small-cell lung cancer. *Journal of the National Cancer Institute,* 83(12):855–861.

Fukuoka, M., Masuda, N., and Ariyoshi, Y. (1996). Therapeutic approach to disseminated small cell lung cancer. In: Aisner J., Arriagada, R., Green, M., et al (eds.). *Comprehensive Textbook of Thoracic Oncology.* (pp. 496–511). Baltimore: Williams & Wilkins.

Fukuoka, M., Niitani, H., Suzuki, A., Motomiya, M., Hasegawa, K., Nishiwaki, Y., Kuriyama, T., Ariyoshi, Y., Negoro, S., Masuda, N., Nakajima, S., and Taguchi, T., for the CPT-11 Lung Cancer Study Group. (1992). A phase II study of CPT-11, a new derivative of camptothecin, for previously untreated non-small cell lung cancer. *Journal of Clinical Oncology,* 10(1):16–20.

Furuse, K., Fukuoka, M., Kawahara, M., Nishikawa, H., Takada, Y., Kudoh, S., Katagami, N., and Ariyoshi, Y. (1999). Phase III study of concurrent versus sequential thoracic radiotherapy in combination with mitomycin, vindesine, and cisplatin in unresectable stage III non-small cell lung cancer. *Journal of Clinical Oncology,* 17(9):2692–2699.

Furuse, K., Kuba, M., Yamori, S., Nakai, Y., Negoro, S., Katagami, N., Takada, Y., Kinuwaki, E., Kawahara, M., Kubota, K., Sakuma, A., and Niitani, H., for the Japan Vinorelbine Lung Cancer Cooperative Study Group. (1996). Randomized study of vinorelbine versus vindesine in previoulsy untreated stage IIIB or IV non-small cell lung cancer. *Annals in Oncology,* 7:815-820.

Furuse, K., Kubota, K., Kawahara, M., Ogawara, M., Kinuwaki, E., Montomiya, M., Nishiwaki, Y., Niitani, H., and Sakuma, A. (1994). A phase II study of vinorelbine, a new derivative of Vinca alkaloid, for previously untreated advanced non-small cell lung cancer. *Lung Cancer,* 11(5–6):385–391.

Gatzemeier, U., Heckmeyr, M., Neuhass, R., Schluter, I., Pawel, J., Wagner, H., and Dreps, A. (1995). Phase II study with paclitaxel for the treatment of advanced inoperable non-small cell lung cancer. *Lung Cancer,* 12(Suppl. 2):101–106.

Gatzemeier, U., Shepherd, F., LeChevalier, T., Weynants, P., Cottier, B., Groen, H., Rosso, R., Mattson, K., Cortes-Funes, H., Tonato, M., Burkes, R., Gottfired, M., and Voi, M. (1996). Activity of gemcitabine in patients with non-small cell lung cancer: A multicenter, extended phase II study. *European Journal of Cancer,* 32A(2):243–248.

Georgoulias, V., Papadakis, E., Alexopoulos, A., Stavrinidis, E., Bania, E., Rapti, A., Grigoratou, T., Kouroussis, C., Kakolyris, S., and Samonis, G. (1999). Docetaxel plus cisplatin versus docetaxel plus gemcitabine chemotherapy in advanced NSCLC: A preliminary analysis of a multicenter randomized phase II trial. *Proceedings of the American Society of Clinical Oncology,* 18:1778.

Ginsberg, R., Hill, L., Eagan, R., Thomas, P., Mountain, C., Deslauriers, J., Fry, W., Butz, R., Goldberg, M., and Waters, P. (1983). Modern thirty-day operative mortality for surgical resections in lung cancer. *The Journal of Thoracic and Cardiovascular Surgery,* 86:654–658.

Goto, K., Nishiwaki, Y., Takada, M., Fukuoka, M., Kawahara, M., Sugiura, T., Kurita, Y., Watanabe, K., Noda, K., Yoshimura, K., Tamura, T., and Saijo, N. (1999). Final results of a phase III study of concurrent vs. sequential thoracic radiotherapy in combination with cisplatin and etoposide for limited stage small cell lung cancer: The Japan Clinical Oncology Group Study. *Proceedings of the American Society of Clinical Oncology,* 18:1805.

Graham, M.V. (2001). NSCLC: Value of three-dimensional conformal radiotherapy: Pro. In: Movsas, B., Langer, C.J., and Goldberg, M. (eds.). *Controversies in Lung Cancer: A Multidisciplinary Approach.* (pp 279–298). New York: Marcel Dekker.

Greco, F. and Hainsworth, J. (1997). Multidisciplinary approach to potentially curable non-small cell carcinoma of the lung. *Oncology,* 11(1):27–36.

Gridelli, C., Perrone, F., Gallo, C., De Marinis, F., Ianniello, G., Cigolari, S., Cariello, S., Di Costanzo, F., D'Aprile, M., Rossi, A., Migliorino, R., Bartolucci, R., Bianco, A.R., Pergola, M., and Monfardini, S. (1997). Vinorelbine is well tolerated and active in the treatment of elderly patients with advanced non-small cell lung cancer: A two-stage Phase II study. *European Journal of Cancer,* 33(3):392–397.

Gridelli, C., Perrone, F., Gallo, C., Rossi, A., Barletta, E., Barzelloni, M., Creazzola, S., Gatani, T., Fiore, F., Guida, C., and Scognamiglio, F. (1999). Single-agent gemcitabine as second-line treatment in patients with advanced non-small cell lung cancer (NSCLC): A phase II trial. *Anticancer Research,* 19(5C):4535–4538.

Hainsworth, J., Hopkins, L., Thomas, M., and Greco, F. (1998). Paclitaxel, carboplatin, and extended-schedule oral etoposide for small cell lung cancer. *Oncology,* 12(Suppl 2):31–43.

Hainsworth, J., Thompson, D., and Greco, F. (1995). Paclitaxel by 1-hour infusion: An active drug in metastatic non-small cell lung cancer. *Journal of Clinical Oncology,* 13(7):1609–1614.

Hainsworth, J., Thompson, D., Urba, W., Hon, J., Thompson, K., Hopkins, L., and Greco, F. (1997). One hour paclitaxel plus carboplatin in advanced non-small cell lung cancer: Results of a Minnie Pearl Cancer Research Network phase II study. *Lung Cancer,* 18(Suppl. 1):23–24.

Hammoud, Z., Anderson, R., Meyers, B., Guthrie, T., Roper, C., Cooper, J., and Patterson, G. (1999). The current role of mediastinoscopy in the evaluation of thoracic disease. *The Journal of Thoracic and Cardiovascular Surgery,* 118: 894–899.

Harwood, K. (1996). Non-small cell lung cancer: An overview of diagnosis, staging and treatment. *Seminars in Oncology Nursing,* 12(4): 285–294.

Jelliffe, R. (1973). Letter: Creatinine clearance: Bedside estimate. *Annals of Internal Medicine,* 79(4):604–615.

Jeremic, B., Shibamoto, Y., Acimovic, L., and Milisavljevic, S. (1997). Initial versus delayed accelerated hyperfraction-ated radiation therapy and concurrent chemotherapy in limited-stage small cell lung cancer: A randomized study. *Journal of Clinical Oncology,* 15(3):893–900.

Johnson, D. and Piantadosi, S. (1994). Chemotherapy for resectable stage III non-small cell lung cancer—Can that dog hunt? *Journal of the National Cancer Institute,* 86(9):650–651.

Johnston, M. (1997). Curable lung cancer: How to find it and treat it. *Postgraduate Medicine,* 101: 155–163.

Katakami, N., Takada, M., Negoro, S., Ota, K., Fujita, J., Furuse, K., Ariyoshi, Y., Ikegami, H., and Fukuoka, M. (1996). Dose escalation study of carboplatin with fixed-dose etoposide plus granulocyte-colony stimu-lating factor in patients with small cell lung carci-noma. *Cancer,* 77(1):63–70.

Kelly, K., Crowley, J., Bunn, P., Livingston, R., and Gandara, D. (1999). A randomized phase III trial of paclitaxel plus carboplatin versus vinorelbine plus cis-platin in untreated advanced NSCLC. A Southwest Oncology Group trial. *Proceedings of the American Society of Clinical Oncology,* 18:1777.

Khuri, F.R., Keller, S.M., and Wagner, H., Jr. (1999). Non-small cell lung cancer and mesothelioma. In: Pazdur, R. and Hoskins, W. J. (eds.). *Cancer Management: A Multidsciplinary Approach* (3rd ed.). Melville, NY: Research and Representation.

Komaki, R. (1985). Preoperative and postoperative irradiation for cancer of the lung. *J Belge Radiology,* 68: 195–198.

Komaki, R., Cox, J., Hartz, A., et al. (1985). Characteristics of long-term survivors after treatment for inoperable carcinoma of the lung. *American Journal of Clinical Oncology,* 8: 362-370.

Kosmidis, P., Samantas, E., Fountzilas, G., Pavlidis, N., Apostolopoulou, F., and Skarlos, D. (1994). Cisplatin/etoposide versus carboplatin/etoposide chemotherapy and irradiation in small cell lung cancer: A randomized phase III study. *Seminars in Oncology,* 21(3, Suppl. 6):23-30.

Koukourakis, M., Bahlitzanakis, N., Froudarakis, M., Giatromanolaki, A., Georgoulias, V., Koumiotaki, S., Christodoulou, M., Kyrias, G., Skarlatos, J., Kostantelos, J., and Beroukas, K. (1999). Concurrent conventionally fractionated radiotherapy and weekly docetaxel in the treatment of stage IIIb non-small cell lung cancer. *British Journal of Cancer,* 80(11):1792-1796.

Kudoh, S., Fujiwara, Y., Takada, Y., Yamamoto, H., Kinoshita, A., Ariyoshi, Y., Furuse, K., and Fukuoka, M. (1998). A phase II study of irinotecan combined with cisplatin in patients with previously untreated small-cell lung cancer. West Japan Lung Cancer Group. *Journal of Clinical Oncology,* 16(3):1068-1074.

Kudoh, S., Kurihara, N., Okishio, K., Hirata, K., Yoshikawa, J., Masuda, M., Takada, M., Takeda, K., Negoro, S., and Fukuoka, M. (1996). A phase I-II study of weekly irinotecan (CPT-11) and simultaneous thoracic radiotherapy (TRT) for unresectable locally advanced non-small cell lung cancer (NSCLC). *Proceedings of the American Society of Clinical Oncology,* 15:372.

Kunitoh, H., Sailo, N., and Nagao, K. (1999). Cisplatin and irinotecan versus cisplatin and vindesine in advanced stage IIIB/IV NSCLC: A multicentric phase II study. Abstracts and Proceedings of ECCO 10.

Kunitoh, H., Watanabe, K., Onoshi, T., Furuse, K., Niitani, H., and Taguchi, T. (1996). Phase II trial of docetaxel in previously untreated, advanced non-small cell lung cancer: A Japanese cooperative study. *Journal of Clinical Oncology,* 14(3):1649–1655.

Lam, S. (1994). Photodynamic therapy of lung cancer. *Seminars in Oncology,* 21(6, Suppl. 5): 15–16.

Langer, C., Gandara, D., Calvert, P., Edelman, M., and Ozols, R. (1999). Gemcitabine and carboplatin in combination: An update of phase I and phase II studies in non-small cell lung cancer. *Seminars in Oncology,* 26(1, Suppl. 4):12–18.

Langer, C., Leighton, J., Comis, R., O'Dwyer, P., McAleer, C., Bonjo, C., Engstrom, P., Litwin, S., and Ozols, R. (1995). Paclitaxel and carboplatin in combination in the treatment of advanced non-small cell lung cancer: A phase II toxicity, response and survival analysis. *Journal of Clinical Oncology,* 13(8):1860–1870.

Langer, C., Manola, J., Bernardo, P., Bonomi, P., Kygler, A., and Johnson, D. (2000). Advanced age alone does NOT compromise outcome in fit non-small cell lung cancer (NSCLC) patients (pts) receiving platinum (DDP)-based therapy (TX): Implications of ECOG 5592. *Proceedings of the American Society of Clinical Oncology,* 19:1912.

Lardinois, D.,Weder, W., Hany, T., Karnel, E., Korom, S., Seifert, B., vonSchulthess, G., and Steinert, H. (2003). Staging of non-small cell lung cancer with integrated positron-emission tomography and computed tomography. *New England Journal of Medicine,* 348 (25): 2500-2507.

Lau, D., Leigh, B., Gandova, D., Edelman, M., Morgan, R., Israel, V., Lara, P., Wilder, R., Ryu, J., and Doroshow, J. (1999). Weekly carboplatin, twice weekly paclitaxel, and thoracic radiation followed by carboplatin/paclitaxel for stage III non-small cell lung cancer. *Seminars in Oncology,* 26(3, Suppl. 2):70.

LeChevalier, T. (1996). Single agent activity of gemcitabine in advanced non-small cell lung cancer. *Seminars in Oncology,* 23:36–42.

LeChevalier T, Arriagada, R., Quoix, E., Ruffie, P., Martin, M., Tarayre, M., Lacombe-Terrier, M., Douillard, J., and Laplanche, A. (1991). Radiotherapy alone versus combined chemotherapy and radiotherapy in non-resectable non-small cell lung cancer: First analyses of a randomized trial in 353 patients. *Journal of the National Cancer Institute,* 83(6):417–423.

LoCicero, J. (2000). Segmentectomy and lesser pulmonary resections. In: Shields, T., LoCicero, J., and Ponn, R. *General Thoracic Surgery,* 5th ed. (pp. 433–438). Philadelphia: Lippincott Williams and Wilkins.

LoCicero, J., Ponn, R. and Daly, B. (2000). Surgical treatment of non-small cell lung cancer. In: Shields, T., LoCicero, J., and Ponn, R. *General Thoracic Surgery,* 5th ed. (pp. 1311–1341). Philadelphia: Lippincott Williams and Wilkins.

Lorusso, V., Carpagnano, F., Frasci, G., Panza, N., Di Rienzo, G., Cisternino, M., Napoli, G., Orlando, S., Cinieri, S., Brunetti, C., Palazzo, S., and De Lena, M. (1995). Results of a clinical multicentric randomized phase II study of non-small cell lung cancer treated with vinorelbine-cisplatin versus vinorelbine alone. *International Journal of Oncology,* 6(1):65-68.

Machtay, M., Seiferheld, W., Komaki, R., Cox, J.D., Sause, W.T., and Byhardt, R.W. (1999). Is prolonged survival possible for patients with supraclavicular node metastases in non-small cell lung cancer treated with chemoradiotherapy?: Analysis of the Radiation Therapy Oncology Group experience. *Int J Radiat Oncol Biol Phys,* 44(4): 847–53.

Manegold, C., Stahel, R., Mattson, K., Ricci, S., van Valree, N., Bergman, R., and ten Bokkel Huinink, W., on behalf of a European multinational study group. (1997). Randomized phase II study of gemcitabine (GEM) monotherapy versus cisplatin plus etoposide (C/E) in patients (pts) with locally advanced or metastatic non-small cell lung cancer (NSCLC). *Proceedings of the American Society of Clinical Oncology,* 16:1651.

Mattson, K., Von Pawel, J., Manegold, C., Postmus, P., and Clarke, S. (1999). MTA (Multitargeted Antifolate, LY231514) in NSCLC patients who failed previous platinum or non-platinum chemotherapy: A phase II trial. *Proceedings of the American Society of Clinical Oncology,* 18:1892.

Marks, L.B. and Sibley, G. (1999). The rationale and use of three-dimensional radiation treatment planning for lung cancer. *Chest,* 1116(6): 539S–45S.

Martin, C., Isla, D., Gonzalez-Larriba, J., Felip, E., Camps, C., Anton, A., Carrato, A., Azagra, P., Alberola, V., Massuti, B., Sanchez, J., Monzo, M., and Rosell, R. (1999). A phase II study of bi-weekly gemcitabine/paclitaxel in advanced non-small cell lung cancer (NSCLC). *Proceedings of the American Society of Clinical Oncology,* 18:1781 (abstr).

Martini, N., Rusch, V., Bains, M., Kris, M., Downey, R., Flehinger, B., and Ginsberg, R. (1999). Factors influencing ten-year survival in resected stages I to IIIA non-small cell lung cancer. *The Journal of Thoracic and Cardiovascular Surgery,* 117: 32–38.

Mehta, M. (1996). Endobronchial radiotherapy for lung cancer. In: Pass, H., Mitchell, J., Johnson, A., and Turrisi, A. (eds.). *Lung Cancer: Principles and Practice,* (pp. 741–751). Philadelphia: Lippincott-Raven.

Miller, V. (1999). Docetaxel (Taxotere) in combination with vinorelbine in non-small cell lung cancer. *Seminars in Oncology,* 26(3, Suppl. 10):12–14.

Miller, V., Rigas, J., Francis, P., Grant, S., Pisters, K., Venkatraman, E., Woolley, K., Heelan, R., and Kris, M. (1994). Phase II trial of docetaxel given at a dose of 75 mg/m2 with prednisone premedication in non-small cell lung cancer. *Proceedings of the American Society of Clinical Oncology,* 13:362.

Millward, M., Bishop, J., and Lehnert, M. (1999). Phase II trial of docetaxel and carboplatin in advanced NSCLC. *Proceedings of the American Society of Clinical Oncology,* 18:1994.

Millward, M., Bishop, J., Friedlander, M., Levi, J., Goldstein, D., Olver, I., Smith, J., Toner, G., Rischin, D., and Bell, D. (1996). Phase II trial of a 3-hour infusion of paclitaxel in previously untreated patients with advanced non-small cell lung cancer. *Journal of Clinical Oncology,* 14(1):142–148.

Murphy, W., Fossella, F., Winn, R., Shin, D., Hynes, H., Gross, H., Davilla, E., Leimert, J., Dhingra, H., Raber, M., Krakoff, I., and Kong, W. (1993). Phase II study of Taxol in patients with untreated advanced non-small cell lung cancer. *Journal of the National Cancer Institute,* 85(5):384–396.

Murphy, W., Winn, R., Huber, M., Fosella, F., Goldberg, D., Presant, C., Flynn, P., Coldman, B., Clements, S., Raber, M., and Hong, W. (1994). Phase II study of taxol (T) in patients (pts) with non-small cell lung cancer (NSCLC): The role of Taxol (TAX). *Proceedings of the American Society of Clinical Oncology,* 13:363.

Murray, N., Coy, P., Pater, J., Hodson, I., Arnold, A., Zee, B., Payne, D., Kostashuk, E., Evans, W., and Dixon, P. (1993). The importance of timing of thoracic irradiation in the combined modality treatment of limited-stage small cell lung cancer. *Journal of Clinical Oncology,* 11(2):336–344.

Murray, N., Livingston, R., Shepherd, F., James, K., Zee, B., Langleben, A., Kraut, M., Bearden, J., Goodwin, J., Grafton, C., Turrisi, A., Walde, D., Croft, H., Osoba, D., Ottaway, J., and Gandara, D. (1999). Randomized study of CODE versus alternating CAV/EP for extensive-stage small-cell lung cancer: An intergroup study of the National Cancer Institute of Canada Clinical Trials Group and the Southwest Oncology Group. *Journal of Clinical Oncology,* 17(8):2300–2308.

National Comprehensive Cancer Network (NCCN). (2003). Practice Guidelines in Oncology, V1 (2003).

Nakai, H., Fukuoka, M., Furuse, K., Nakao, I., Yoshimori, K., Ogura, T., Hara, N., Sakata, Y., Saito, H., and Hasegawa, K. (1991). An early phase II study of CPT-11 for primary lung cancer. *Gan To Kagaku Ryoha* [Japanese Journal of Cancer and Chemotherapy], 18(4):607–612.

Nakai, H., Takada, M., Yokoyama, A., Negoro, S., Kurita, Y., Fukuoka, M., and Niitani, H. (1994). Results of phase II studies of gemcitabine in patients with non-small cell lung cancer in Japan. *Lung Cancer,* 11(Suppl. 1):120.

Negoro, S., Fukuoka, M., Niitani, H., Suzuki, A., Nakabayashi, T., Kimura, M., Motomiya, M., Kurita, Y., Hasegawa, K., and Kuriyama, T. (1991). A phase II study of CPT-11: A camptothecin derivative in patients with primary lung cancer. *Gan To Kagaku Ryoha* [Japanese Journal of Cancer and Chemotherapy], 18:1013–1019.

Non-Small Cell Lung Cancer Collaborative Group. (1995). Chemotherapy in non-small cell lung cancer: A meta-analysis using updated data on individual patients from 52 randomized clinical trials. *British Medical Journal,* 311(7010):899–909.

Optivus Technology, Inc. (2001). What is proton beam therapy? *www.optivus.com*–accessed on 9/27/01.

Pazdur, R., Coria, L., Hoskins, W., and Wagman. (2003). *Cancer Management: A Multidisciplinary Approach,* 6th edition. PRR, Melville, N.Y.

Perng, R., Chen, Y., Ming-Liu, J., Tsai, C., Liu, W., Yang, K., and Whang-Peng, J. (1997). Gemcitabine versus the combination of cisplatin and etoposide in patients with inoperable non-small cell lung cancer in a phase II randomized study. *Journal of Clinical Oncology,* 15(5):2097–2102.

Pfeiffer, P., Sorenson, P., and Rose, S. (1995). Is carboplatin and oral etoposide an effective and feasible regimen in patients with small cell lung cancer? *European Journal of Cancer,* 31A:64–69.

Ramanathan, R. and Belani, C. (1997). Chemotherapy for advanced non-small cell lung cancer: Past, present, and future. *Seminars in Oncology,* 24(4):440–454.

Ranson, M., Davidson, N., Nicolson, M., Falk, S., Carmichael, J., Lopez, P., Anderson, H., Gustafson, N., Jeynes, A., Gallant, G., Washington, T., and Thatcher, N. (2000). Randomized trial of paclitaxel plus supportive care versus supportive care for patients with advanced non-small cell lung cancer. *Journal of the National Cancer Institute,* 92(13):1074–1080.

Ranson, M., Jayson, G., Perkins, S., Anderson, H., and Thatcher, N. (1997). Single agent paclitaxel in nonsmall cell lung cancer: Single center study using a 3-hour administration schedule. *Seminars in Oncology,* 24(Suppl. 12):12–16.

Rapp, E., Pater, J., Willan, A., Cormier, Y., Murray, N., Evans, W., Hudson, D., Clark, D., Feld, R., and Arnold, A. (1988). Chemotherapy can prolong survival in patients with advanced non-small cell lung cancer: Report of a Canadian multicenter randomized trial. *Journal of Clinical Oncology,* 6(4):633–641.

Reed, C. and Silvestri, G. (2000). Diagnosis and staging of lung cancer. In: Shields, T., LoCicero, J., and Ponn, R. *General Thoracic Surgery,* 5th ed. (pp. 1297–1309). Philadelphia: Lippincott Williams and Wilkins.

Reilly, J. 1999. Evidence-based preoperative evaluation of candidates for thoracotomy. *Chest,* 116. pp. 474–476.

Rice, T.W., Adelstein, D.J., Ciezki, J.P., Becker, M.E., Rybicki, L.A., Farver, C.F., Larto, M.A., and Blackstone, E.H. (1998). Short-course induction chemoradiotherapy with paclitaxel for stage III non-small cell lung cancer. *Ann Thorac Surg,* 66(6):1909–14.

Richards, F., White, D., Muss, H., Powell, B., Cruz, J., Andes, A., Spell, N., Tarassoff, P., and Matt, J. (1994). Phase I trial of gemcitabine over 30 minutes in patients with non-small cell lung cancer. *Proceedings of the American Society of Clinical Oncology,* 13:344.

Rinaldi, M., Della Giulia, M., Venturo, P., Del Medico, P., Serrone, L., Capomolla, E., and Lopez, M. (1994). Vinorelbine as single agent in the treatment of advanced NSCLC. *Proceedings of the American Society of Clinical Oncology,* 13:360.

Roth, B., Johnson, D., Einhorn, L., Schacter, L., Cherng, N., Cohen, H., Crawford, J., Randolph, J., Goodlow, J., and Broun, G. (1992). Randomized study of cyclophosphamide, doxorubicin, and vincristine versus etoposide and cisplatin versus alternation of these two regimens in extensive small cell lung cancer: A phase III trial of the Southeastern Cancer Study Group. *Journal of Clinical Oncology,* 10(2):282–291.

Rothe, J., Grammer, S., Swisher, S., Nemunaitis, J., Merritt, J., and Meyn, R. (2000). Gene replacement strategies for treating non-small cell lung cancer. *Seminars in Radiation Oncology,* 10(4):333–342.

Salazar, A. and Westcott, J. (1993). The role of transthoracic needle biopsy for the diagnosis and staging of lung cancer. *Clinical Chest Medicine,* 14:99.

Sause, W., Scott, C., Taylor, S., Johnson, D., Livingston, R., Komaki, R., Emami, B., Curran, W., Byhardt, R., and Turrisi, A. (1995). Radiation Therapy Oncology Group (RTOG) 88-08 and Eastern Cooperative Oncology Group (ECOG) 4588: Preliminary results of a phase III trial in regionally advanced unresectable non-small cell lung cancer. *Journal of the National Cancer Institute,* 87(3):198–205.

Scalliet, P., Goor, C., Galdermans, D., Van Meerbek, J., Groen, H., Van der Leest, A., Westerink, H., Jungnelius, U., and Turrisi, A. (1998). Gemzar (gemcitabine) with thoracic radiotherapy—a phase II pilot study in chemonaive patients with advanced non-small cell lung cancer (NSCLC). *Proceedings of the American Society of Clinical Oncology,* 17:1923.

Schiller, J., Harrington, D., Belani, C., Langer, C., Sandler, A., Krook, J., Zhu, J., and Johnson, D. (2002). Comparison of four chemotherapy regimens for advanced non-small-cell lung cancer. *New England Journal of Medicine,* 346(2):92-98.

Sekine, I., Nishiwaki, Y., Watanabe, K., Yoneda, S., Saijo, N., and the East Japan Paclitaxel Study Group. (1996). Phase II study of 3-hour infusion of paclitaxel in previously untreated non-small cell lung cancer. *Clinical Cancer Research,* 2(6):941–945.

Shepherd, F., Burkes, R., Cormier, Y., Crump, M., Feld, R., Strack, T., and Schulz, M. (1996). Phase I dose-escalation trial of gemcitabine and cisplatin for advanced non-small cell lung cancer: Usefulness of mathematic modeling to determine maximum-tolerable dose. *Journal of Clinical Oncology,* 14(5):1656–1662.

Shepherd, F., Dancey, J., Ramlau, R., Mattson, K., Gralla, R., O'Rourke, M., Levitan, N., Gressot, L., Vincent, M., Burkes, R., Coughlin, S., Kim, Y., and Berille, J. (2000). Prospective randomized trial of docetaxel versus best supportive care in patients with non-small-cell lung cancer previously treated with platinum-based chemotherapy. *Journal of Clinical Oncology,* 18(10): 2095-2103.

Shields, T. W. (2000). General features of pulmonary resections. In: Shields, T., LoCicero, J., and Ponn, R. *General Thoracic Surgery,* 5th ed. (pp. 375-384). Philadelphia: Lippincott Williams and Wilkins.

Silvestri, G., Tanoue, L., Margolis, M., Barker, J., and Detterbeck, F. (2003). The non-invasvie staging of non-small cell lung cancer. *Chest,* 123(1): 147-156.

Skarin, A., Jochelson, M., Sheldon, T., Malcolm, A., Oliynyk, P., Overholt, R., Hunt, M., and Frei, E. 3rd. (1989). Neoadjuvant chemotherapy in marginally resectable stage III M0 non-small cell lung cancer: Long-term follow-up in 41 patients. *Journal of Surgical Oncology,* 40(4):266-274.

Socinski, M. and Steagal, A. (1997). Phase II trial of 96 hour paclitaxel infusion in patients with non-small cell lung cancer failing previous platinum based or short duration paclitaxel therapy. *Proceedings of the American Society of Clinical Oncology,* 16:1735.

Spiridonidis, C., Laufman, L., Jones, J., Rhodes, V., Wallace, K., and Nicol, S. (1998). Phase I study of docetaxel dose escalation in combination with fixed weekly gemcitabine in patients with advanced malignancies. *Journal of Clinical Oncology,* 16(12):3866-3873.

Sugarbaker, D., Herndon, J., Kohman, L., Krasna, M., and Green, M. (1995). Results of cancer and leukemia group b protocol 8935: A multi-institutional phase II trimodality trial for stage IIIA(N2) non-small cell cancer. *Journal of Thoracic and Cardiovascular Surgery,* 109(3):473–485.

Tan, Flaherty, Kazerooni, and Iannettoni. (2003). The Solitary Pulmonary Nodule. *Chest.* 123(1):895-965.

Tan, V., Herrera, C., Einzroj, A., and Wiernik, H. (1995). Taxol is active as a 3 hour or 24 hour infusion in non-small cell lung cancer. *Proceedings of the American Society of Clinical Oncology,* 14:366.

Tester, W., Jin, P., Reardon, D., Cohn, J., and Cohen, M. (1997). Phase II study of patients with metastatic non-small cell carcinoma of the lung treated with paclitaxel by 3-hour infusion. *Cancer,* 79(4):724–729.

Thomas, M., Rhbe, C., Semik, M., von Eiff, M., Freitag, L., Macha, H., Wagner, W., Klinke, F., Scheld, H., Willich, N., Berdel, W., and Junker, K. (1999). Impact of preoperative bimodality induction including twice-daily radiation on tumor regression and survival in stage III non-small cell lung cancer. *Journal of Clinical Oncology,* 17(4):1185–1193.

Tubiana, M. and Eschwège, F. (2000). Conformal radiotherapy and intensity-modulated radiotherapy. Clinical data. *Acta Oncologica,* 39(5):555–67.

Van Putten, J., Fokkema, E., Smeets, J., and Groen, H. (1999). Phase II study of high-dose epirubicin and gemcitabine in patients with advanced NSCLC. *Proceedings of the American Society of Clinical Oncology,* 18:487.

Veronesi, A., Crivellari, D., Magri, M.D., Cartei, G., Mansutti, M., Foladore, S., and Monfardini, S. (1996). Vinorelbine treatment of advanced non-small cell lung cancer with special emphasis on elderly patients. *European Journal of Cancer,* 32A(10):1809-1811.

Wain, J., Kaiser, L., Johnstone, D., Yang, S., Wright, C., Friedberg, J., Feins, R., Heitmiller, R., Mathisen, D., and

Selwyn, M. (2001). Trial of a novel synthetic sealant in preventing air leaks after lung resection. *The Annals of Thoracic Surgery,* 71: 1623–1629.

Yokoyama, A., Kurita, Y., Watanabe, K., Negoro, S., Ogura, T., Nakano, M., Minoda, S., Niitani, H., and Taguchi, T. (1994). Early phase II clinical study of RP56976 (docetaxel) in patients with primary pulmonary cancer. *Gan To Kagaku Ryoha* [Japanese Journal of Cancer and Chemotherapy], 21(15):2609–2616.

Weisenburger, T. (1994). Effects of postoperative mediastinal radiation on completely resected stage II and III epidermoid cancer of the lung. LCSG 773. *Chest,* 106S: 297–301.

Zehr, K., Dawson, P., Yang, S., and Heitmiller, R. (1998). Standardized clinical care pathways for major thoracic cases reduce hospital costs. *Annals of Thoracic Surgery,* 66:1–6.

Zwitte, M., Cufer, T., and Wein, W. (1999). Phase II trial of gemcitabine and vincristine for stage IV NSCLC. *Proceedings of the American Society of Clinical Oncology,* 18:529.

PART III

Symptom Management

11

Acute Side Effects: Interventions and Teaching

Introduction

❖ Many factors determine the severity of radiation therapy side effects. Symptom management depends on where the radiation therapy beams are aimed.

❖ Acute effects arise during the period when the patient is receiving treatment.

❖ Factors that influence the occurrence and severity of side effects include the:

   1. *Size and location of the treatment field*– Radiation therapy targets the tumor or the tumor bed plus surrounding tissue that may contain microscopic disease or lymph nodes.

   2. *Total dose of radiation therapy prescribed*–The higher the total dose, the greater the tissue damage.

3. *Other tissues or organs in the treatment field*—Sensitive organs could include the esophagus causing esophagitis.

4. *Daily dose of radiation therapy*—Treatments given in large daily doses that shorten the overall treatment time have more acute side effects than lower-dose treatments administered over a longer period of time.

5. *Type of ionizing particles used for treatment*—Electron activity occurs mostly on the skin surface, causing more of a skin reaction than photons, which deeply penetrate the tissue and spare the skin the radiation dose.

6. *Concurrent treatment*—Combination of chemotherapy and radiation therapy potentates the toxicities.

7. *Comorbid diseases*—Individuals with diabetes or who have lupus erythematous and other collagen vascular disease may experience different skin reactions as they could heal slower, which may require that their treatment be interrupted.

Acute Symptomology/Interventions

❖ Although the purpose of radiation is to destroy cancer cells, it also injures normal cells and produces acute side effects.

❖ Acute toxicities occur during the course of irradiation or within 1 month after the completion of therapy.

❖ The potential acute side effects with possible management strategies when treating the thorax with external irradiation are:

1. *Cough*—75% of the patients already have a cough prior to RT and 40% have a severe cough (Chao, Perez, and Brady, 1999). However, cough may increase during treatments and become more productive as radiation opens obstructed airways. Eventually, respiratory mucosa becomes dry and the cough becomes nonproductive. Individuals may be concerned that the increase in cough means that the therapy is not working when indeed the opposite may be true. Coughing may be an extremely debilitating symptom and can lead to a loss of appetite, sleep, and strength.

   ❖ *Management strategies*—If coughing disrupts the ability to eat, rest, or sleep, initial management may be simple over-the-counter cough suppressants with dextromethorphan, i.e. Robitussin DM® (dextromethorphan + Guaifenesin), 2 teaspoons every 4 hours, as needed. If that is not effective, advance to Tessalon Perles® 100mg every 8 hours (max 6 perles/day) and then to a narcotic-containing cough suppressant, as needed: Codeine or Robitussin® with codeine, 1 teaspoon every 3 hours; Hydrocodone/Hycodan,® 5mg every 4 hours; or Hycotuss with guaifenesin, 5-15 cc every 4 hours (max 30cc/day); if cough is severe take Hydromorphone/Dilaudid® 2mg every 3 hours.

❖ *Patient teaching*—Increase fluids when cough becomes productive, especially if tenacious sputum; observe for signs of respiratory infection or tumor lysis.

2. *Dyspnea*—Breathlessness is a problem commonly encountered with advanced lung cancer. It is an unpleasant sensation that can be frightening and can increase an individual's fatigue. It is caused by both the disease and treatment factors.

❖ *Management strategies*—Simple breathing exercises and positioning techniques may help focus the person and relieve dyspnea (purse breathing/bending up and over a table). Oxygen therapy may be offered if oxygen saturation is below 88% before Medicare or other third-party insurance pays for oxygen in the home. Relaxation and coping strategies—music therapy, meditation, guided imagery—can be used for breathing distraction. Pharmaceutical steroids may alleviate the symptoms (prednisone 40mg initially and later taper or Decadron® 16mg a day and taper). Opiods administered through nebulizers may relax the person: Morphine 10mg tablet dissolved in 3 cc of Normal Saline, every 4 hours, prn- side effect may cause bronchospasms, therefore have 2.5 mg albuterol available (Chandler, 1999).

❖ *Patient teaching*—Conservation of energy techniques to decrease the burden on the cardiopulmonary system. Guided imagery and relaxation tapes (free tape from Roche Laboratories—Music for Radiation Therapy by Belleruth Naparstek).

3. *Pharyngitis/esophagitis*—Esophagitis is the major dose-limiting side effect of thoracic irradiation. Epithelial cells of the pharynx and esophagus are highly radiosensitive and are frequently within the treatment area for lung cancer. Even with conformal treatment planning and treatment delivery, a portion of the esophagus receives a significant radiation dose during pulmonary irradiation.

Pharyngitis and esophagitis usually occurs 2-3 weeks into treatment or after 20–30 Gy. If pain develops prior to this, suspect thrush or gastroespohageal reflux. With esophagitis, individuals can feel a lump or fullness in their throat and have difficulty or very painful swallowing. Certainly the combination of chemotherapy and radiation may increase the incidence of esophageal injury.

❖ *Management strategies*—For radiation induced esophagitis, initially begin with liquid aloe rinses on the first day of therapy, i.e. Radiocare Oral Rinse® (Carrington product) or Oral

Magic® (MPM Medical). Some practitioners would prefer to use Carafate® Slurries instead (1 tablet (1 gram) in 1 tablespoon of water, dissolve and swallow). Then, if pain develops after 2 weeks, mucosal anesthetics and agents to coat irritated surfaces may be helpful, i.e. Triple Mix of Benadryl, Maalox, and Xylocaine, or Miracle Mouth Wash—which adds mycostatin, hydrocortisone, and tetracycline to the mixture. If pain is unrelieved or worsens then add prn systemic pain medications (i.e. hydrocodone and acetaminophen/Lortab Elixir,® 15 cc every 4 hours, prn), or scheduled long acting pain medications (Oxycontin,® MS Contin,® or transdermal patches—Duragesic® patches). Again, words of wisdom, don't forget obvious other causes of sore throat, i.e. Thrush (simply treated with fluconazole or ketoconazole). Also, research is in progress with the use of cytoprotective agents and decreasing esophagitis with amifostine (Senzer, 2002). Cytoprotection from receiving Ethyol® (amifostine) is reported to reduce the incidence of chemoradiation-induced esophagitis (Leong, 2003; Movsas, 2003, and Antonadou, 2002). While Ethyol® has not received FDA approval for this indication, several clinical trials have provided evidence that pre-treatment with Ethyol® reduces the incidence of esophagitis without affecting antitumor efficacy of radiation treatment in advanced lung cancer (Antonadou, 2001). The

most recent Phase III study, RTOG 98-01 conducted by Movsas (2003), confirmed that
Ethyol® is a dose-and-schedule-dependent drug
and from patients' perspective, utilizing a daily
self-assessment swallowing log, there was sta-
tistical significance shown at the end of treatment in reducing esophagitis. Refer to the
studies identified above for dosage.

❖ *Patient teaching*–Important dietary counseling: soft, non-spicy foods, no acidic
foods/drinks, and no alcohol. High caloric,
high protein diets are important for weight
maintenance and quicker healing time in
recovery period. Encouragement to stop
smoking is helpful in the initial consult, but
not always realistic during treatment.
Unfortunately, smoking is an irritant and
retards healing.

4. *Weight loss/anorexia*–Any or all of the symptoms just mentioned can contribute to poor
appetite. At least 50% of patients with lung
cancer have been reported as experiencing
some weight loss during the 6 months prior to
diagnosis (weight loss ≥ 2 pounds/week or ≥
10% of their initial weight occurs). Anorexia
has been reported in 60% of patients by the
fourth week of treatment.

❖ *Management strategies*–If available, a nutritional consultation with a dietician can individ-
ualize a plan to maintain and, if possible, gain

weight. Dietician reviews the person's protein and caloric intake, identifies any areas requiring improvement, and recommends specific dietary modifications to help patients maintain good nutrition during therapy. Pharmacological approaches can be initiated early:

I. Over-the-counter appetite stimulants:
   a. Eldertonic®, 1 tablespoon, three times a day
   b. Ginger capsules, 1 capsule three times a day
   c. Zinc (improves taste), 18-45mg, three times a day

II. Medication options for anorexia:
   a. Megace®, 800mg, every day (20cc)
   b. Marinol®, 2.5 mg, twice a day (before lunch and supper), max. 20mg daily
   c. Decadron®, 1.5 mg once a day (increasing to 2mg, three times a day)

❖ *Patient teaching*–Inverted food pyramid applies during therapy. Individuals eating less because of decreased appetite or esophagitis, need foods that are rich in protein and calories. For the treatment and recovery period, no restrictions are placed on fat or oil intake. Once swallowing starts to become difficult, avoiding hard or rough foods, heavily seasoned food or spices, extremes in temperatures, and avoiding beverages with alcohol, high acid content, or carbonation will help lessen severity of discomfort. Eating 6-7 small meals a day is preferred over 3 square meals a day. Nutritional supplements should be included, such as Nestle Sweet Success®, Instant Carnation Breakfast®, Ensure Plus®, Boost Plus®, Shandishake®, or other high calorie milkshakes. Eating Hints is a helpful booklet, and is free of charge from the American Cancer Society. If administering Ethyol®, hydration is very important, although nausea, vomiting, and hypotension are less common via subcutaneous route vs. intravenously. Injection-site and systemic allergy reactions appear to be more common when given subcutaneously. Teach patients to report any skin irritation or rash.

5. *Skin changes*—Radiation-induced skin reactions are a function of fractional dose, total dose, and fractionation schemes. Normal progression is erythema, dry desquamation, to moist desquamation. Most patients treated for thoracic irradiation do not progress to the moist desquamation stage. The main goal of managing early radiodermatitis is maintenance of intact epithelium, primarily by minimizing scratching or rubbing of the damaged tissue. Pruritus can often occur too.

❖ *Management strategies*—Where skin is entacted, hydrogels or emollient moisturizers are recommended. Examples of hydrogels, containing aloe vera, are Radiocare Gel® (Carrington) or RadiaPlex RX Gel® (MPM

Medical). However, in Phase III randomized trials, applying aloe vera has not been shown to protect against radiation damage. Other creams are available; for example, Biafine®, Eucerin®, or TheraCare®. Emollients like Aquaphor® provide excellent moisture barriers. Applying a moisturizer prior to a radiation treatment may actually intensify the reaction, therefore instruct individuals not to put anything on one hour prior to treatment. If a pruritic rash develops, try steroidal cream; for example, Diprolene® 0.05% cream, applying it sparingly twice a day until the rash has resolved or no longer pruritic. After completion of treatment, a zinc-based product can be recommended to aid in healing.

❖ *Patient teaching*—Skin care would include washing with mild soap without deodorant or perfumed soaps and lukewarm water, using only the recommended creams/lotions, not scrubbing off any markings, protecting area from sun exposure, and not using direct heating pads or hot water bottles.

6. Pain—Pain related to lung cancer may be due to tumor compression of an organ structure, direct nerve compression, bone erosion, or brain metastasis (headaches). Also, patients experience pain caused by treatment induced tissue reactions (mucositis, esophagitis, pharyngitis, dry and moist desquamation)

❖ *Management strategies*—In-depth pain algo-rithms can be found in:

I. Internet link sites:

 ❖ NCCN National Comprehensive Cancer Network, *www.nccn.org*

 ❖ NCCN Practice Guidelines for Cancer Pain, *http://www.partnersagainstpain. com/html/profed/pmc/pe_pmc2.htm?pg= 6271&section=pe_pmc2*

 ❖ American Pain Society, *http://www.ampainsoc.org/*

 ❖ Agency for Healthcare Research and Quality: Acute Pain Management Guidelines and Management of Cancer Pain Guidelines, *http://hstat.nlm.nih.gov/hq/Hquest/db/ local.arahcpr.arclin.capc/screen/ DLTocDisplay/s/45378/action/DLToc*

 ❖ American Alliance of Cancer Pain Initiatives, *www.aacpi.org*

II. Reference books (Resources: US Department of Health and Human Services Quick Reference Guide for Clinicians: Management of Cancer Pain: Adults).

 ❖ Some clinical pearls are:

 ❖ Learn about the relative efficacy of any prescribed pain medications and their dosing frequency.

❖ Assess on the universal 0 to 10 scale (0=no pain and 10=worst pain imaginable), prior and after intervening.

0-2 rating, choose non-opioid analgesics

3-5 rating, choose Class III or possibly IV narcotics

>6 rating, choose Class II narcotics

❖ Short acting pain medications indicated every 4-6 hours and long-acting pain medications indicated every 12 hours. Remember to provide a short-acting medication along with long-acting for rescue or breakthrough pain. Adding NASIDs may be helpful for more chronic pain.

❖ Begin a stool regime when first ordering narcotics. Increasing fluids and fiber in diet will be helpful.

7. *Radiation pneumonitis*—The incidence and severity of this response is related to the volume of lung irradiated, total dose and fractionation, and concomitant chemotherapy. It manifests by dry cough, low-grade fevers, and dyspnea approximately 8-12 weeks after completion of radiation therapy (Chao, Perez, and Brady, 1999). Several clinical trials have shown promising results with administration of Ethyol®, in preventing radiation pneumonitis (Roychowdhury, 1999: Gopal, 2001, Gopal, 2003).

   ❖ *Management strategies*—Bedrest and NSAID, (Ibuprofen, Naprosyn®, or Indocin®) are generally recommended along with some bronchodilators. Antibiotics are not indicated until there is associated secondary infection. However, some patients may develop severe dyspnea and require hospitalization and steroid therapy.

❖ *Patient teaching*–Typically, this is transient and does not require treatment. Supportive care may be required and does not necessarily mean the lung cancer is growing.

8. *Hoarseness*–This symptom presents because of radiation-induced cough or compression of the recurrent laryngeal nerve by central tumors or mediastinal lymphadenopathy.

❖ *Management strategies*–Initially the symptom management should focus on resting the voice as much as possible and treatment of the pharyngitis. Alternative methods of communication (such as note writing) should be encouraged. Hopefully, if the cause is due to compression, radiation treatment will soon shrink the tumor and relieve the pressure, allowing a more normal voice sound.

9. *Fatigue*–Fatigue is the number one reported acute symptom experienced by radiation therapy patients (60%) and the longest-lasting side effect experienced by cancer patients. Fatigue is a complex, multifactoral problem that develops over time even prior to therapies, manifesting as decreased motivation or interest; feelings of sad-

ness, frustration, or irritability; and decreased cognitive abilities and depression. Patients with advanced disease usually present with weight loss, anorexia, pain, and dyspnea, which can all contribute to fatigue as well. Fatigue can start two weeks after starting radiation therapy to the chest. It may gradually increase as therapy continues, however, it does not necessarily mean the cancer is getting worse.

The etiology and underlying mechanisms of cancer-related fatigue are not well understood, although an interaction of multiple mechanisms is likely and further research in this area is warranted. Fatigue can be attributed to the waste products that result from tumor breakdown or to the nutritional requirements of the tumor. Energy is also rapidly depleted by the increased metabolic rate accompanying tumor growth or infection (Piper, 1998).

* Management strategies—Assessment is key to the recognition and management of cancer-related fatigue. A number of validated and reliable tools are available to assess fatigue in patients with cancer: Piper Fatigue Scale, Functional Assessment of Cancer Therapy-Fatigue (FACT-F), and Brief Fatigue Inventory. In 2000, the National Comprehensive Cancer Network (NCCN) published guidelines for the assessment and management of cancer-related fatigue.

Non-pharmacological strategies improving fatigue include: exercise (walking or light swimming), restorative therapy (active/passive ROM exercises), good nutrition, adequate sleep by establishing regular bedtimes and waking-up times, having a conducive sleep environment (use for sleep only, not watching TV or reading), relaxing and avoiding stressful interactions before sleep, and avoiding caffeine, nicotine, alcohol, and exercise 4 hours before bedtime. Pharmacological approaches include correcting anemia with biological erythropoietin (Procrit®), psychostimulants (methylphenidate, Pemoline®, dextroamphetamin), or low-dose corticosteroid (dexamethasone or Prednisone®).

❖ *Patient teaching*—Using assessment tools regularly helps medical caregivers identify the presence of fatigue, as well as develop a standardized intervention plan to help manage the symptoms. The overall goal of these guidelines is to ensure that all lung cancer individuals who experience fatigue will be identified and treated promptly and effectively. Evaluation is focused on predisposing factors/etiologies like pain, depression, anemia, sleep disorder, and other conditions.

Understanding cancer-related fatigue and learning methods for how to conserve energy, using distraction (music, guided imagery), and learning stress management techniques are important for the nurse to teach patients.

a. Internet Resources:

❖ Oncology Nursing Society (ONS), *www.ons.org*

❖ National Comprehensive Cancer Network (NCCN), *www.nccn.org/patient_gls/_english/_fatigue/index.htm*

❖ CancerFatigue, *www.cancerfatigue.org*

10. *Depression*—More insidious than physical symptoms of lung cancer, but perhaps more devastating for patients with lung cancer, is depression. Depression during end-of-life care may be variable and can be difficult to treat to the patient's or family's satisfaction.

❖ *Management strategies*—Pharmacological and psychiatric therapy may be of great value for patients with depression and their families. The four major classifications are tricyclics, heterocyclics, selective serotonin reuptake inhibitors (SSRIs), and monoamine oxidase inhibitors (MAOIs). Selection of medication should be individualized. Selection should be based on possible drug interactions, the individual's age, and adverse effects (SSRIs do not have the anticholinergic, antihistaminic, or alpha-adrenergic receptor blocking activity of tricyclics).

❖ *Patient Teaching*—Explaining to patients that depression is a very common symptom experienced by many lung cancer patients, and encouraging support groups or providing pastoral support can help through difficult times. Light exercise appears to have both direct and indirect effects on relief of depression.

11. *Cerebral edema due to brain metastases*—CNS changes can occur if the lung cancer has spread to the brain. The tumor and cerebral edema can be very problematic, causing numerous side effects.

    ❖ *Management strategies*—If the patient has CNS symptoms, start immediately on Decadron® (10mg IV), then 4mg, orally, four times a day to help alleviate symptoms of weakness, confusion, visual disturbances, headaches, nausea/vomiting, and others. Remember to add antacids to help with the gastric distress and anti-hypnotics if the patient develops insomnia.

    ❖ *Patient Teaching*—Reinforcement of potential side effects of steroids and encouraging individual to inform health professionals of problems are both important.

12. *Nausea and vomiting*—In the era of multimodalities, the increasing use of chemoradiation increases the intensity of the toxicities. Typically in the past, this was not a common symptom when treating thoracic irradiation, but with concurrent chemotherapy, nausea and vomiting may occur with chemotherapy agents (cisplatin, vinblastine).

a. *Management strategies*—pharmacological agents include:

❖ Primary medications options:

Compazine® 10mg, (p.o.) 1 tablet every, 6 hours, prn

Compazine® 25 mg (suppository), 1 suppository, twice a day, prn

Compazine® 5mg/5 ml (liquid), 1-2 teaspoons every 6 hours, prn

Ativan® 1 mg (p.o./subl.), 1 tablet every 6 hours, prn

Reglan® 10mg, 1 tablet every 6 hours, prn

Phenergan® 25 mg (p.o.) 1 tablet every 4-6 hours, prn

❖ Secondary medication options:

Zofran® 8mg, 1 tablet or ODT every 8 hours, prn

Marinol® 2.5- 5.0 mg, 1 tablet three to four times a day

Kytril® 1 mg, 1 tablet, twice a day, prn

Steroids

❖ Consider laboratory tests (electrolytes/CBC) and intravenous fluids for hydration.

❖ *Patient teaching*—Avoid greasy, fatty foods; eat in small amounts; use aromatherapy (peppermint); try drinking ginger tea (Kuebler and Esper, 2002).

12

Late Side Effects: Interventions and Teaching

Introduction

❖ Late or chronic complications of radiation therapy are defined as complications occurring or persisting 90 days or later after the completion of treatment.

❖ When radiation therapy is carefully planned and delivered with respect to normal tissue tolerances, severe late complications are not routinely seen. Dose guidelines for the total volume of lung treated, as well as doses to the spinal cord, heart, and esophagus, must be considered. When these dose limits (based on 1.8-2.0 Gy per fraction) are respected, the risk of severe complications, such as cardiomyopathy or myelitis, is less than 55% at 5 years after therapy.

❖ Long-term side effects are more directly related to

the dose per fraction than to the total radiation dose. The risk of more intense late complications increases as the dose per fraction increases.

Late symptomology/interventions

❖ The chronic toxicities or long term effects can include:

1. *Radiation fibrosis of the lung*—Fibrosis is a permanent response to the lung tissue reaction that occurs during radiation therapy and most patients do not experience clinical symptoms related to the fibrosis. However, those who were already compromised may experience chronic dyspnea, cough, and increased sensitivity to pollutants and irritants.

   ❖ *Management strategies*—A specific treatment for fibrosis is not available, and the focus should be on individual respiratory symptom management.

2. *Esophageal stricture or stenosis*—Stenosis, ulceration, and fistula formation are typically rare. Evaluation for esophageal dilatation may be necessary.

   ❖ *Management strategies*—Individualized depending on degree of injury and symptoms.

3. Hoarseness—May result from permanent nerve injury/damage.

   ❖ *Management strategies*—Frequently rest the

voice, avoid singing and long periods of consistent use. Pain medications typically are not required.

4. *Skin changes including alopecia*–Patients who receive > 5000cGy to the chest may experience hyperpigmentation and alopecia of the skin within the treatment fields. Mild fibrous of the skin may occur.

    ❖ *Management strategies*–Typically nothing is required. Keeping skin moisturized and avoiding direct sunlight is recommended.

5. *Cardiac sequella*–Relatively rare, but pericardial effusion, constrictive percarditis, and cardiomyopathy can happen.

    ❖ *Management strategies*–Professional healthcare monitoring is required. Caution is required with certain chemotherapeutic agents, such as doxorubicin (synergistic cardiotoxicity).

6. *Spinal cord myelopathy*–Care is taken to ensure total spinal cord dose, length of cord irritated, and the fractionation schedule to avoid any spinal cord damage.

    ❖ *Management strategies*–It is extremely important to recognize spinal cord compression and treat as an emergency.

7. *Brachial plexopathy*–Depends if the supraclavical area is involved. Patients present without pain, but with edema and signs of upper trunk

(C-5 through C-7) dysfunction. When associated with lymphedema, the symptoms of the brachial plexopathy may improve with treatment of the lympedema.

* *Management strategies*–May include nerve blocks, cordotomy, rhizotomy, or oral narcotic management for uncontrolled chronic pain.

Documentation

* Evidence-based medicine requires quality documentation and is an important step in the process (Watkins, Bruner, Moore, Higgs, Haas, 2001). By documenting and publishing interventions and clinical outcomes, our strides towards an evidence-based practice model will be accomplished.

* The NCI Toxicity Criteria Version 3, with the input from the Radiation Therapy Oncology Group (RTOG) and European Organization for Research and Treatment of Cancer (EORTC) Acute Effects Criteria Instrument, provides scales for many different organ systems and symptoms. This is a very useful tool for grading the severity of acute and long term effects.

* Also, the Radiation Therapy Patient Care Record: A Tool for Documenting Nursing Care is an excellent resource for radiation therapy personnel (ONS, 2002). These site-specific documentation

tools provides a weekly assessment and grading of severity of acute effects of radiation therapy in all sites, including lung cancer, utilizing most of the NCI's toxicity scales.

Follow-up

❖ Surveillance of lung cancer patients after initial treatment depends on the response to treatment.

❖ Suggested follow-up evaluation should be performed every 3 months for a minimum of 3 years, then every 6 to 12 months for the next 2 years, then annually (Chao, Perez, and Brady, 1999).

❖ The evaluation should include:
   ❖ Complete history and physical examination
   ❖ Careful visual inspection and physical examination of the chest and regional lymphatic system
   ❖ Chest X-ray
   ❖ Laboratory studies: CBC, electrolytes, BUN, creatinine, and liver function studies
   ❖ Any additional studies that would depend on presenting symptoms or abnormal physical or radiographic findings

13

Key Clinical Implications of Symptom Management Interventions

Summary of Acute and Late Symptomology

❖ To summarize, the acute and long-term side
   effects for lung tumors are:
   (Liebel and Phillips, 1998; Perez and Brady1998).

Acute	Long term
cough	lung fibrosis
dyspnea	esphageal stenosis
pharyngitis/esophagitis	permanent hoarseness
weight loss/anorexia	permanent hoarseness
skin change	permanent skin changes
pain	cardiac sequella
pneumonitis	spinal cord myelopathy
hoarseness	brachial plexopathy

<u>Acute (cont.)</u>

fatigue

depression

cerebral edema (brain mets)

nausea/vomiting

❖ Despite an incredible amount of effort, lung cancer statistics for the twentieth century are still frightening and depressing.

❖ Although there has been an explosion of knowledge in the biology of lung cancer and a better understanding of risk factors for lung cancer, improvements in the five-year survival rates have been minimal.

❖ Nevertheless, there is some optimism. The challenges still remain of how to best treat the patient and manage their symptoms.

References: Chapters 11–13

Antonadou, D., et al. (2001). Randomized Phase III trial of radiation treatment ± amifostine in patients with advanced stage lung cancer. *International Journal Radiation Oncology, Biology, Physics,* 51:915-922.

Antonadou, D., et al. (2002). Radiotherapy or chemotherapy followed by radiotherapy with or without amifostine in locally advanced lung cancer. *Seminars Radiation Oncology,* 12 (1):50-58.

Chandler, S. (1999). Nebulized opioids to treat dyspnea.

The American Journal of Hospice and Palliative Care, Jan:418-422.

Chao, K., Perez, C., and Brady, L. (1999). *Lung Cancer. Radiation Oncology: Management Decisions.* Philadelphia: Lippincott-Raven.

Gopal, R., et al. (2001). The effects of radiation therapy, chemotherapy and the radioprotector amifostine on the diffusion capacity of patients with non-small cell lung cancer. ASTRO Abstract #33.

Gopal, R., et al. (2003). The relationship between local dose and loss of function for irradiated lung. *International Journal of Radiation Oncology, Biology, Physics,* 56:106-113.

Kuebler, K., and Esper, P. (2002). *Palliative Practices from A-Z for the Bedside Clinician.* Pittsburgh, PA: ONS.

Leog, S., et. al. (2003). Randomized double-blind trial of combined modality treatment with or without amifostine in unresectable stage III non-small cell lung cancer. *Journal of Clinical Oncology,* 21:1767-1774.

Liebel, S. and Phillips, T. (1998). *Textbook of Radiation Oncology.* Philadelphia: W.B. Saunders.

Movsas, B., et al. (2003). Phase III study of amifostine in patients with locally advanced non-small cell lung cancer (NSCLC) receiving intensive chemo/hyperfractionated radiation. Radiation Therapy Oncology Group RTOG 98-01. Proceedings at American Society of Clinical Oncology (ASCO Abstract #21814)

Perez, C. and Brady, L. (1998). *Principles and Practice of Radiation Oncology,* 3rd Edition. Philadelphia: Lippincott-Raven.

Piper. (1997). Fatigue Mechanisms in Cancer Patients: Developing Nursing Theory. *Oncology Nursing Forum,* 14(6):17-23.

Roychowdhury, E., et al. (1999). A phase II trial of amifostine with paclitaxel, caroplatin, and concurrent radiation therapy for unresectable non-small cell lung cancer. Proceedings at American Society Clinical Oncology (ASCO) Abstract #15688.

Senzer, N. (2002). A phase III randomized evaluation of amifostine in stage IIIA/IIIB non-small cell lung cancer patients receiving concurrent carboplatine, paclitaxel, and radiation therapy followed by gemcitabine and cisplatin intensification: Preliminary findings. *Seminar in Clinical Oncology,* Dec. 29(6 Supp 19):38-41.

Watkins-Bruner, D., Moore-Higgs, G., and Haas, M. (2001). *Outcomes in Radiation Therapy: Multidisciplinary Management.* Sudbury, Massachusetts: Jones and Bartlett.

PART IV

Evidence-Based Guidelines, Clinical Trials, and Resources

14

Evidence-Based Guidelines

Introduction

❖ Originating from evidence-based medicine (EBM), evidence-based practice (EBP) is the process of basing clinical decisions on research findings and the best available evidence rather than intuition and traditional standards of the past.

❖ EBP "defines care that integrates best scientific evidence with clinical expertise, knowledge of pathophysiology, knowledge of psychosocial issues, and decision making preference of the patients" (Rutledge and Grant, 2002).

❖ Outcomes-based management, a method of measuring, evaluating, and improving care, leads to EBP (Watkins-Bruner, Moore-Higgs, and Haas, 2001).

❖ The EBP's multidisciplinary approach involves:

1. Identifying the patient problem (can evolve from patient care, quality improvement teams, or professional clinical experience).

2. Searching for the evidence (refer to different levels of evidence and resources).

3. Critically analyzing the evidence (based on merit, feasibility, and utility).

4. Synthesizing all the evidence and extracting pertinent information as it applies to the problem and making a practice recommendation (setting specific or organizational systems).

5. Implementing the recommendations and changing clinical guidelines.

6. Evaluating the effectiveness of recommendations and continually monitoring process (ONS Evidence-Based Practice Resource Center, 2001; Cope, 2003).

Types of evidence

❖ Types of evidence can range from the highest level of scientific clinical research to the non-research evidence of the opinion and experience of the healthcare provider. The hierarchy should be identified to the participants and cited in any recommendations.

❖ The levels of evidence are:

Hierarchy of Levels of Research

Research Based Evidence	*Strength of Evidence*
Meta-analysis/systematic review of multiple controlled clinical trials	Strongest
Experimental studies, such as well-controlled randomized clinical trials	
Systematic reviews of all types of research	
Multiple non-experimental studies, including descriptive, correlational, and qualitative research	
Published evidence-based practice guidelines, for example, by professional organizations	

Non-research Based Evidence

Case studies through benchmarking or systematically obtained	
Program evaluation, quality improvement data, or case reports	
Regulatory or legal opinions	
Opinions of experts-standards of practice, practice guidelines	Weakest

(Rutledge, D. and Grant, M., 2002)

Guidelines resources

❖ Resources available online to assist in EBP are:

1. Agency for Healthcare Research and Quality,
   www.ahcpr.gov

2. Cochrane Database of Systematic Reviews,
   www.update-software.com/
   cochrance/abstract.htm

3. National Guidelines Clearinghouse,
   www.guideline.gov

4. National Comprehensive Cancer Network (NCCN),
   http://www.nccn.org/index.html

5. NCI/PDQ Non-small Cell Lung Cancer
   Treatment and Small Cell Lung Cancer
   Treatment, Enter lung cancer in the search box
   and then select Lung Cancer Home Page.
   Contains expert reviewed summaries about the
   treatment of NSCLC and SCLC.
   http://cancer.gov

Other Evidence-Based Resources For Lung Cancer

http://www.ahrq.gov/clinic/epcix.htm
   Evidence Reports from Agency for Health Care
   Research and Quality

http://oncology.medscape.com
   Medscape Lung Cancer Resource Center

http://www.nlm.nih.gov/medlineplus/lungcancer.html
   MEDLINEplus Health Information Lung Cancer

15

Clinical Trials

Introduction

❖ In 2001, the National Cancer Institute (NCI) had
  approximately 50 different clinical trials regis-
  tered for the treatment of lung cancer, with radiotherapy either alone or in combination with a
  systemic or surgical modality. Of these, the
  majority (33) are for NSCLC. The majority of the
  trials were being conducted by the NCI or one of
  the cooperative groups, including the Radiation
  Therapy Oncology Group (RTOG) or the European
  Organization for the Treatment of Cancer
  (EORTC). Others were being conducted by either
  single or multi-institutional groups. The focus of
  the trials appeared to be on the following:

  1. What is the value of altered-fraction and
     3D-CRT in the treatment of NSCLC?

  2. What is the optimal sequencing of radiother-
     apy with various chemotherapy agents?

3. What is the role of treatments such as photo-dynamic therapy in combination with endo-bronchial brachytherapy?

4. What is the role of other systemic therapies such as biologicals and complementary therapies?

5. What is the efficacy of agents that can reduce the toxicity of radiotherapy, thus allowing dose escalation?

❖ It has been established that novel radiotherapy administration schedules and techniques as well as chemotherapy regimens for combined modality therapy are essential for improving the management of lung cancer. A number of Phase I and Phase II randomized trials of new chemoradiation regimens are currently enrolling patients. In addition, trials with adjuvant monoclonal antibodies, shark cartilage extract, and photodynamic therapy are being conducted.

Clinical Trials Resources

❖ Clinical trials offer lung cancer individuals the best opportunity to receive the most up-to-date, aggressive treatments available. Unfortunately, there is no single resource for locating clinical trials for lung cancer. Emerging studies are continually updated.

1. NCI Clinical Trials
   Toll free telephone: 1-800-4CANCER
   Web site: *http://www.nci.nih.gov*

2. NIH/NLM Clinical Trials
   888-FIND-NLM (888-346-3656)
   Web site: *clinicaltrials.gov*

3. Centerwatch Clinical Trials Listing Service
   Customer Service: 800-765-9647
   Web site: *www.centerwatch.com*

4. Clinical Trials Resources (Lung Cancer Online)
   Web site:
   www.lungcanceronline.org/clinical.htm

5. Radiation Therapy Oncology Group (RTOG)
   Web site: *www.rtog.com*

6. Eastern Cooperative Oncology Group (EGOG)
   Web site: *http://ecog.dfci.harvard.edu*

7. Southwest Oncology Group (SWOG)
   Web site: *http://swog.org/*

8. North Central Cancer Treatment Group
   (NCCTG)
   Web site: *http://ncctg.mayo.edu/*

16

Resources

Introduction

❖ Making informed decisions is the cornerstone for
lung cancer patients and their families. Numerous
materials are available to assist in making these
critical decisions. These are excellent resources for
health professionals, individuals, families, and
friends.

Lung Cancer Organization

The following chart identifies available organizations that can assist patients and their families.

Organization	Mission
1. Alliance for Lung Cancer Advocacy, Support and Education (ALCASE) 1601 Lincoln Ave. Vancouver, WA 98660 Toll free telephone: 1-800-298-2436 Web site: *http://www.alcase.org* E-mail: info@alcase.org	A non-profit organization offering educational information, phone buddy support system, newsletters, and information searches that can improve the quality of lives of individuals with lung cancer.
2. American Cancer Society (ACS) National Office 1599 Clifton Road NE Atlanta, GA 30329 Toll free telephone: 1-800-ACS-2345 Web site: *http://www.cancer.org*	A nationwide, community-based organization that focuses on cancer advocacy, education, and research activities. Local state-wide chapters are available.
3. American Lung Association (ALA) 1740 Broadway, 14th Floor New York, NY 10019 Toll free telephone: 1-LUNG USA Web site: *http://www.lungusa.org*	A national organization that promotes lung health, focusing on preventing lung cancer with an emphasis on tobacco cessation, environmental health issues effecting lung cancer, and lung co-morbidities, for example asthma and chronic obstructive lung disease.

Organization	Mission
4. National Cancer Institute (NCI) Office of Cancer Communications Room 10A24, Building 31 9000 Rockville Pike Bethesda, MD 20892 Toll free telephone: 1-800-4CANCER Web site: *http://www.cancer.gov*	A national governmental organization that offers up-to-date research information on lung cancer, including prevention, diagnosis, and treatment. Supports computerized Physicians Data Query (PDQ) identifying the latest types of cancer treatments and clinical trials.
5. National Comprehensive Cancer Network (NCCN) 50 Huntingdon Pike, Suite 200 Rockledge, PA 19046 Toll free telephone: 1-888-909-NCCN Web site: *http://www.nccn.org*	A not-for-profit corporation that is an alliance of the world's leading cancer centers. Established in 1995 to enhance the leadership role of member institutions in the evolving managed care environment, the NCCN seeks to support and strengthen the mission of member institutions in three basic areas: 1.) To provide state-of-the-art cancer care to the greatest number of patients in need, 2.) To advance the state-of-the-art in cancer prevention, screening, diagnosis, and treatment through excellence in basic and clinical research, and 3.) To enhance the effectiveness and efficiency of cancer care delivery through the ongoing collection, synthesis, and analysis of outcomes data.

Internet Sites for Lung Cancer

❖ When using the Internet, it is extremely important to recognize and evaluate creditable Web sites. The following sites have been evaluated by the Oncology Nursing Society's three critical criteria: credibility of the information provider, disclosure of sponsorship, and privacy of data collected from users (Clark and Gomez, 2001).

Web Sites	Organization
http://www.aarc.org	American Association for Respiratory Care
http://gek.bestvwh.net	American Heart and Lung Institute
http://www.cancercareinc.org	Cancer Care
http://www.cancernews.com/lung.htm	Cancer News on the Net: Lung Cancer
http://www.meds.com/lung/lunginfo.html	The Lung Cancer Information Center
http://www.ons.org	Oncology Nursing Society: Lung Cancer (under special projects)

Screening

❖ Another easily accessible Web site offering a free screening questionnaire, fact sheet, and risk list is the Harvard School of Public Health. They have developed their own Web site "Harvard Center for Cancer Prevention", which estimates an individual's risks for lung cancer, among other types of cancers, and provides personal tips on prevention. Support groups are also found on the Internet for education and advocacy.

http://www.yourcancerrisk.harvard.edu

Complementary and Alternative Medicine (CAMS)

1. American Academy of Medical Acupuncture
   http://www.medicalacupuncture.org
   Professional site with articles on acupuncture, a list of frequently asked questions, and acupuncturist locator.

2. National Center for Complementary and Alternative Medicine (NCCAM)
   http://nccam.nih.gov
   Offers information on complementary and alternative medicine therapies, including NCI/PDQ expert reviewed fact sheets on individual therapies and dietary supplements.

3. NCI Office of Cancer Complementary and Alternative Medicine (OCCAM)
   http://www.cancer.gov/occam
   A clearinghouse for NCI's CAM activities.

References: Chapters 14–16

Clark, P. and Gomez, E. (2001). Details on demand: Consumers, cancer information and the Internet. *Clinical Journal of Oncology Nursing,* 5(1):19-24.

Cope, D. (2003). Evidence-based practice: Making it happen in your clinical setting. *Clinical Journal of Oncology Nursing,* 7(1):97-98.

ONS EBP Online Resource Center "Evidence Search" Section, *http://onsopcontent.ons.org/toolkits/ebp/ process_model/evidence_search/evidence_search.htm.*

Rutledge, D. and Grant, M. (2002). Introduction. *Seminars in Oncology Nursing,* 18(1): 1-2.

Watkins-Bruner, D., Moore-Higgs, G., and Haas, M. (2001). *Outcomes in Radiation Therapy.* Sudbury, Massachusetts: Jones and Bartlett.

Index

Page numbers followed by *t* denote tables.